# THE ABC's of WOMEN'S HEALTH

## What Every Woman Needs to Know

### By

W9-BYH-727

### Sylvia M. Barchue, RN, MS

### Betty L. Gadson, RN

*"A woman's health is her capital."*
Harriet Beecher Stowe

# THE ABC's of WOMEN'S HEALTH

## What Every Woman Needs to Know

By

Sylvia M. Barchue, RN, MS

Betty L. Gadson, RN

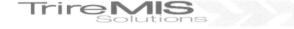

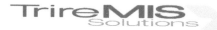

Published by TrireMIS Solution, LLC Norwalk, CT, USA.
Copyright © 2021 Sylvia M. Barchue, RN, MS; Betty L. Gadson, RN
Copyright Registration Number: TXu 2-279-776

*ISBN: 978-0-9820767-0-5*

*McLean Enterprise Cover Design by Mark Lambertson. Printed in the USA.*

# CONTENTS

## INTRODUCTION

My sisters, this book is written solely for you. It deals only with the female. And while some diseases and illnesses affect both male and female, we think it's important to concentrate specifically on the unique set of issues women face.

We are both Registered Nurses, who for years have been advocates for family members and friends unfamiliar with the medical field and have little experience dealing with healthcare providers. We have often seen people struggle to understand their own bodies and how certain diseases might impact their lives. Our goal here is to educate you because frankly, you deserve no less. As the title "A, B, C's" indicates, we deal with these diseases and conditions alphabetically. Of course, this book is not exhaustive, and we do not claim to have covered all that the female needs to know.

Our attempt is to address issues / diseases in basic terms that everyone can understand.

This book is meant to be both entertaining and factual, therefore we have interjected some humour here and there to lighten the mood. And finally, we have added some helpful health maintenance tips in the "Nuts & Bolts" section at the end of the book.

So read through "The ABCs of Women's Health" for yourself and recommend it to all of your friends, including the men for the ladies in their lives. Women are the caregivers and nurturers for the entire family. Finally, a book focused on their needs so they can continue to be healthy and able to be the backbone of the family.

*Betty and Sylvia*

## DISCLAIMER

This book is not intended to be used as a medical guide for self-diagnosis. Please see your doctor for regular check-ups as well as when feeling ill.   It is intended for use as a reference only. It does not replace the need to seek medical attention when necessary. Please always follow the instructions, guidance and treatment plan that may be provided by your Primary Care Physician (PCP).

## FOREWORD

*In October 2015, I was at a photo shoot in Long Island City, NY wondering why I was there. My plans were to drop off my sister Sonia to the photo shoot, then to go to Queens, NY to have breakfast with an 'adopted' sister June and hang out at her home; then pick Sonia up later in the day. When we got to the photo shoot, we realized that logistically it made sense for me to just stay there.*

*So, here I was at this photo shoot with about 4 to 6 hours of wait time and nothing to do or eat. Well, I have an energy bar which is a poor substitute for the expected good solid Caribbean breakfast at June's. And, I have my laptop. I usually travel with more magazines than I can read on the road, but I was on my way to breakfast and to hang out with June, I did not expect to be 'stranded' at the photo shoot.*

*How did I spend my time?*

*Well, I had promised to write a foreword for my sister Sylvia's new book, and I had my laptop, so I set about writing this foreword.*

*What did I write about?*

*I looked around the makeup and wardrobe room and looked at my beautiful sister Sonia as she applied her makeup.*

*Inspiration…… I wrote about this beautiful woman, who will have been in a vegetative state or dead when she became ill. By the grace of God and due to the guidance of our sister, Sylvia, who had had many years of medical care knowledge and training. Sylvia made educated decisions on Sonia's behalf about her care at a very desperate time due to the fact that she was Sonia's health care proxy.*

*I started to type, and the words flowed.*

*Here goes.......*

*Just as financial health is very important to women of all ages, so is, or should be physical health.*

*We grew up in an age where we took physical health for granted, thinking we would always be healthy. We were entitled to good health, forever. Right?*

*However, as we have aged and taken care of children and more so parents, we now realize that good health is not automatic. We have to work for it. At this time, we need to understand our bodies, what make things work well, how to respect and maintain our bodies, and how to care for our loved ones.*

*Therefore, in an effort to maintain our physical health, we need to start with the basics.*

*A great first step to understanding these basics is by reading 'The ABCs of Women's Health.'*

*I am very proud of my sister, Sylvia Barchue, and her friend Betty Gadson, for sharing their years of healthcare experience, insights, and expertise.*

*I am particularly proud of Sylvia, who also authored, 'My Sister, My Friend, My Miracle,' upon the recovery of our sister Sonia, who had brain surgery as treatment for an AVM. An AVM is an Arteriovenous malformation, which is an abnormal connection between arteries and veins that can be silent or bleed or lead to other serious medical problems; and possibly death.*

*I became particularly, though reluctantly, interested in health care when Sonia had a cerebral haemorrhage from the AVM. For example, before this, I did not know that the muscles in the buttocks were what propelled and managed the science of walking. I understood this when Sonia was paralyzed on one side and had to learn to walk again. I had to work with her on many* evenings when the therapist had either left or did not work that day.

Caring for a loved one leaves one, at least left me, and other non-medical caretakers in a state of dependence, possibly near panic, with heavy dependence on the medical staff. My family was blessed to have our own medical consultant in Sylvia. When the doctor in charge of Sonia's care was ready to clip an aneurysm, I was ready to sign on the dotted line. Sylvia, on the other hand, authoritatively told the doctor that you do not clip an AVM, which Sonia had. She proceeded to tell him how an AVM is treated. This was the very first time that our family received the respect due from the doctor. Sylvia immediately took Sonia out of that doctor's care, and, before virtual medical care became a norm, Sylvia implemented this in Sonia's care.

Sonia continued treatments to stabilize her at Norwalk Hospital, Connecticut, but her treatments were guided by a doctor in California who had copies of all of her X-rays, CT scans, Angiogram and MRIs; and held frequent conference calls with Sylvia. This California doctor passed Sonia's care onto his associate who at this time was at Yale University Hospital, and had previously worked under his direction. Additionally, the California doctor was at that time the foremost authority on AVMs in the USA.

Sonia went on to have brain surgery at Yale New Haven Hospital, Connecticut and has since fully recovered to the point where she earned an MA degree in government and a JD (law degree), travelled the world on many missionary trips and actually taught business at a university in China for a year.

I write all of the above to emphasize the need for the understanding of our bodies in this age when many of us will become caretakers, planned and unplanned, cheerfully or reluctantly.

*I lacked the necessary knowledge when decisions had to be made about Sonia's care. Thank God that we had Sylvia in the family who could make the educated decisions. And thank God for Sonia's miraculous response and subsequent recovery to be a fully functioning adult. God perfectly orchestrated the people and places for Sonia's ultimate recovery to full functionality.*

*Our story ended happily. Therefore, I wish all of the readers of this book, good health for yourselves and your families, and happy endings to your health challenges.*

*My sister and friend, Sylvia and Betty, may God continue to bless you as you bless others through this and future books. I am in awe of the medical profession and all of the professionals who care for us and our loved ones. I also give you applause.*

*With utmost respect,*

*Stacia Morris*

## TESTIMONIALS

*While I am currently a physician at a Veteran's Hospital where the majority of patients are male, I have taken care of many women in my career; and as a female, women's issues, whether it is social, political, or health-related, interest me. Furthermore, I am frequently confronted by friends and co-workers/colleagues, usually female, with questions about health, health care, and disease. The questions posed are sometimes personal, sometimes basic, and sometimes serious. I can understand how some may feel uncomfortable in discussing various concerns with an unfamiliar healthcare provider, especially if it does not pertain to you or it truly is a "simple" matter. This is why I find resources like "The ABC's of Women's Health" helpful, but I also hope it gives you the courage to go to and to trust your healthcare provider because we DO understand. Take advantage of resources such as "ABC's" and those listed for more information to educate yourself. I too often see women take care of themselves last, attending to their family and friends first. You are the best self-advocate. Most importantly, take care of yourself, feel good about yourself; you will see and feel the difference. You are worth it!*

*Bindu Raju, MD, FCCP*
*Pulmonary and Critical Care Medicine*
*Director ICU, James J Peters VA Medical Center*
*Assistant Professor, Icahn School of Medicine at Mount Sinai;*
*Assistant Clinical Professor, Columbia University School of Medicine.*

*"Extremely easy to understand, very basic and informative."*

*Zinoba Khan, MD*
*Internal Medicine/Pulmonary/Critical Care/ Sleep Medicine*
*Physician ICU, James J. Peters VA Medical Center*

*What a great resource for women everywhere! An easy to read and simple guide to all the beautiful ins and outs of the female body, mind, and spirit. I hope women everywhere will share this resource with all of their friends and use it as a motivator and reminder to put ourselves first! To the best of health, balance and harmony to women all around the world!*

*Priscilla Aponte, EdD,MSN,RN-BC*
*Director of Nursing*
*Community Living Center*
*James J Peters VA*
*130 West Kingsbridge*
*Bronx, NY*


## ACKNOWLEDGEMENTS

There are some special women in our lives who we will like to thank for helping to make this book a reality. I would like to give a special 'Thank You' to my mother and mentor, Constance 'Connie' Morris, the strongest, most courageous and consistent prayer warrior that I have known. She is resting in peace.

Additionally, I would like to acknowledge the following women for their continuous support, guidance and demonstration of love through editing, formatting, design and general support of making this book possible.

These women are:
Elsa Alfred, Luz Mark, Jozeyl Morris, Sherry-Ann Morris, Stacia Morris, Sonia Morris Pollard , Jackie Washington
Thanks also to Bindu Raju, MD; Zinoba Khan, MD; Priscilla Aponte, EdD, MSN & RNBC; for reading the book and providing testimonials.

# ABDOMEN

## Introduction

The Abdomen is better known as the "tummy" or "belly". The tummy /belly is normally soft until pregnancy occurs. Also, during the menstrual cycle, you will experience cramps or feeling bloated.

The tummy/belly stretches during pregnancy as the fetus or baby grows and it is possible to develop stretch marks.

If for any reason you have prolonged tummy / belly pain or you notice that your tummy / belly is bigger than normal or looks and feels bloated, you must contact your doctor.

As you grow older the tummy/belly gets round or bigger, most often due to abdominal muscle weakness and fat. In order to avoid this eat a healthy diet and exercise. Please be sure to include strength training as well as cardiovascular exercise.


# AIDS

## (Acquired Immune Deficiency Syndrome) or HIV (Human Immunodeficiency Virus)

### Introduction

This disease got more recognition when many famous people became infected with the virus that causes the disease. Until then, not much attention was given to the disease.

### How one contracts HIV / AIDS

Usually HIV / AIDS is transmitted by sexual contact, by injecting illegal drugs into the veins with dirty needles, or through blood transfusions when a blood donor is infected.

The number of people infected with HIV / AIDS through blood transfusions has declined due to the improvement in screening and the testing of blood samples.

When someone is diagnosed with HIV / AIDS, do not isolate the person. It is at this time emotional support is needed since HIV / AIDS carries stigma and prejudices. Instead, educate yourself about the disease so that you can remain safe while becoming a better support.

HIV / AIDS can be passed from a mother to her baby in the womb or at birth. It passes by the breast milk to the baby and can sometimes be fatal to an infant.

Signs and Symptoms
Signs and Symptoms may be absent for a long time. Most people seek medical attention when their glands become swollen. This is due to the suppression of the immune system by the virus, which affects the body's ability to fight infections.

Some other Signs and Symptoms are:
- Fatigue
- Fever
- Night sweats
- Weight loss

Diagnosis
HIV / AIDS is diagnosed either by testing blood, saliva, or cells from the inside of the cheek.

The individual should share this diagnosis with their partners so that they can be tested.

Treatment(s)
Knowledge and research of this disease have contributed to improved treatment(s) and management, which have led to a decrease in deaths.

Due to increased awareness, friends and family have been more understanding and supportive of those who have contracted HIV / AIDS.

Usual treatments are:
- Anti-viral Drugs
- Frequent follow ups with the medical practitioner

## ANOREXIA

Introduction

Anorexia (an-oh-REK-see-uh) nervosa is an eating disorder that causes people to obsess about their weight, body image and the foods they eat. Those diagnosed with this disorder make every effort to keep their weight below what is normal for other people in their age group. In order not to gain weight they often starve themselves or eat and then force themselves to vomit the stomach contents.

Anorexia nervosa can lead to death if the person does not receive the help, and support of family and friends to encourage them onto the path of wellness.

This disease is usually well hidden by the sufferer. Once family and friends become aware of this, their support and love are very important to assist in seeking help and changing habits.

Too often in society, we admire others who are slimmer than we are. Models were encouraged to remain slim, but recently we see that there are now many models who do not fit the traditional mold. They are well rounded and are not size 2/4/6, but 12-14 and above and looking good!

<u>Signs and Symptoms</u>
- Constantly exercising / weighing themselves
- Constipation
- Dehydration
- Dizziness
- Excessive weight loss
- Fainting
- Fatigued
- Forced vomiting after meals
- Increase use of laxatives and/ or enemas
- Insomnia
- Irritability /Mood swings
- Preoccupation with food
- Persistently counting calories
- Reduced interest in sex
- Social withdrawal

<u>Seek medical advice</u>

Seek medical advice if / when you have a combination of the above signs and symptoms. Talk to your family and friends to get the support necessary to address this challenge.

<u>Tests / Diagnosis</u>
- Blood work
- Other necessary tests and exams as determined by your doctor
- Physical evaluation
- Physiological examination
- Urine tests
- X-rays

# ARTHRITIS

## Introduction

Arthritis is inflammation in one or more joints, which causes pain, stiffness, swelling, and restricts movement. It affects all ages.

## Causes

Arthritis involves the breakdown of cartilage. Cartilage protects the joints and helps in smooth painless movement. But when there is little or none, the bones rub together, causing pain, swelling and stiffness which may mean that there is inflammation in the joints.

Sometimes the inflammation goes away after treatments by antibiotics. In some cases, a chronic form of arthritis develops.

We can all attest to hearing family and friends complain of arthritis, we have seen the deformed fingers, hear the moaning of pain and complaints of stiffness. Some people say they even know when it is going to rain because the arthritic hands and fingers flare up. Some people have moved to warmer climates to avoid the winter months.

## Signs and Symptoms
- Decreased joint movement /Joint swelling
- Pain / Stiffness

## Tests
- Blood tests / X-rays

## Treatment(s)
- Adjust eating habits
- Exercise (Be careful here, not too strenuous)
- If overweight make all attempts to lose weight
- Medications

# B

# BACTERIAL VAGINOSIS

## Introduction

Bacterial vaginosis (BV) is when the bacteria in the vagina becomes abnormal. You may notice vaginal discharge with a fishy smell. This discharge can be either watery grey or white.

Most women with (BV) have no signs and symptoms. You should seek medical advice when there is a fishy smell or whitish color on your undergarments. To prevent BV, it is recommended that you stop the use of vaginal deodorant, scented soaps and avoid douching.

## Treatment(s)
- Antibiotics
- Stop the use of vaginal deodorant, scented soaps and avoid douching.

# BARTHOLIN'S GLANDS

## Introduction

The Bartholin glands are small and are on either side of the lips of the vagina. These provide secretion during sex. The fluid travels down the ducts and if the ducts become blocked, they form a cyst.

# BARTHOLIN'S CYST

## Introduction

A Bartholin cyst is a small fluid filled sac, which is inside the opening of the vagina. It is common and is usually small and painless. But, it can grow, collect fluids and become painful.

A woman with a Bartholin cyst finds it difficult to walk and have a burning sensation when passing urine.

When to see a Doctor:

You should seek medical advice if / when there is a lump in your vagina area.

## Diagnosis:

- Sample of fluids is sent to the lab for testing
- Tissue is sent to the lab to check for cancer

## Treatment(s)

Usually none.

Other options:

- Anti-inflammatory drugs
- Apply a warm gauze to the area
- Drainage of the cyst
- Warm soaks in the bathtub

## BRCA

## BREAST CANCER (BRCA) GENE TEST

### Introduction

This is a breast cancer gene test. The blood sample checks for specific changes in the genes that help to control the growth of normal cells. This test is done mainly for people with a strong family history of breast or ovarian cancer, and sometimes for those who already have had one of these diseases.

The genes can come from either parent. Recently there have been numerous reports of women and some of them well-known actresses who chose to have this test done and have also had mastectomies and other surgical procedures to eliminate the possibility of having either breast or ovarian cancer.

## BREAST

### Introduction

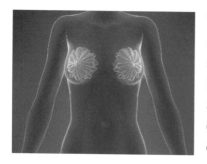
The breasts are found on both sides of the chest wall. They should be examined monthly for lumps, changes in color, shape and size. If you feel a lump in either breast you MUST see your doctor immediately.

Some people are not comfortable doing a self- breast examination; ask your husband or partner if you have one, to do so. Many women report that it is their husband/ partner who first discovered the lump. A lump in the breast does not mean that it is cancerous; there can be many other reasons for this such as: Fibroadenoma, infection, cysts, traumatic fat necrosis or fibrocystic changes (These will be elaborated and explained later).

Visit your gynecologist every year. A breast examination is a part of this visit.

Both breasts should generally look the same. In some people, it may be normal to have one breast smaller or larger than the other. You should contact your doctor immediately if you notice any of the following:

- Changes in the breast size
- Dimpling
- Fluid (if the nipple is squeezed)
- Pain

Breastfeeding is a natural process, but there are many mothers who choose not to breastfeed.

Breast Implants are a matter of choice too!

Also, as we get older the breasts begin to sag. And oh! How we hate this!

## BREAST CANCER

### Introduction

The removal of a breast is a traumatic and emotional experience. Many women pride themselves in having large, well-rounded breasts, and often joke about the flat-chested woman. So, when it becomes necessary to remove a breast the cosmetic issue is a difficult one. The decision for a mastectomy is one that is made with a lot of soul-searching.

Once the decision is made to have the breast removed then it is necessary to obtain the services of a surgeon who specializes in breast surgery. After the surgery is performed, there can be swelling and pain at the operated site.

After the surgery is done you might have a simple drain in your breast for a while to remove any excess fluid. Speak to your healthcare provider about managing your pain since this aids in comfort and assists in an easier post-op recovery. Currently, in preparation for breast reconstruction, a decision may be made to insert an expander during surgery.

After a mastectomy (discussed later), emotional support is needed from family and friends. There are also many support groups available in most communities and it is recommended that you join one. If you join one, it is strongly suggested that your caregiver or partner attend the meetings with you. Studies show that black women develop breast cancer earlier than any other race.

## BREASTS DENSITY

### Introduction

The breasts are dense during puberty and again as you get older. Breast density is a build up of fat in the breasts. On a mammogram this looks like fatty tissue; dense breasts make it difficult to detect cancer since the fatty tissue looks white, just like cancer cells. When breasts are dense, further examination is necessary and your doctor will most likely request a sonogram (ultrasound) or Magnetic Resonance Imaging (MRI).

Dense breasts are staged from:
      Level 1 – almost all fatty tissue
      Level 2 – scattered area of dense tissue, mostly fatty
      Level 3 – mixed dense and fatty tissue
      Level 4 - extremely dense

When a previously normal breast shows density on a mammogram it may be reported to your State Health Department.

Historically, we were told that once breasts density occurred, that this diagnosis never changed. However, this understanding has changed since there have been reports that exercises can change the density of breasts, and a later mammogram can show a normal reading.

Women with dense breast are encouraged to still have an annual mammogram along with a sonogram (ultrasound). You must pay attention to this yourself and if your doctor forgets to order the sonogram (ultrasound) insist that this is done. Remember, we are our own health advocate!

## BREASTS IMPLANTS

### Introduction

Breasts implants are like prostheses. They are used to alter the size and shape of a woman's breasts. They are called a variety of things, but most commonly a 'boob job.' This is done for cosmetic reasons when a woman feels her breasts are either too small or too large; also for breast reconstruction after a mastectomy, or to correct congenital chest deformities. This is also done when there is a male-to-female sex change.

# BREAST SELF EXAMINATION

## Introduction

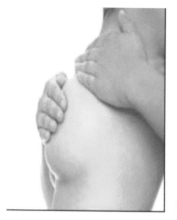 Many of us enjoy looking at ourselves in the mirror. So, strip down, look at your breasts, look at them from every angle you can. Are they nice and well rounded, are they big enough? How often does a woman moan "My breasts are too small, I wish I can get pregnant because as people say the breasts gets bigger when you are pregnant."

Well, look at them now, feel them, do you feel a lump? Are the nipples indented? Is there a discharge? Are they painful? Do they look the same as when you checked them last?

Lie on your bed, right arm above your head. Using your left fingers, press firmly all around your breast. Change hands and repeat the process on the left. If you feel a lump on either side, contact your doctor immediately.

# BREAST SURGERY

## Introduction

Breast surgery is performed for two main reasons:
- Breast cancer - Please refer to the previous section on Breast Cancer
- Cosmetic - to increase or decrease size for personal or health reasons

## Preparing for Breast surgery

This can be a very emotional time because you know that your breast(s) are going to be removed. Also, there is a constant rotation of visits to medical practitioners, surgeons, oncologist (if breast surgery is for cancer) etc.

The following are very important decisions:
- Choosing the best recommended doctors and facility
- The commencement of counselling
- Therapeutic considerations which include chemotherapy and / or radiation

## BULIMIA

### Introduction

Bulimia is a common eating disorder. People with bulimia eat a large amount of food in a short time period, called binging. They will get rid of the food by placing their fingers in the mouth as far back into the throat as they can go, which makes them vomit, called purging.

### Causes
- Family history of bulimia
- Fear of obesity
- Lifestyle
- Wanting to fit in socially

### Signs and Symptoms
- Constant referral to weight loss and body shape
- Forcing yourself to vomit
- Frequent eating binges
- Obsessed with exercising
- Using laxatives, enemas, or diuretics (water pills)
- Visits the bathroom immediately after eating

- Will not eat with other people, eats alone

Bulimia is different from anorexia nervosa which is another eating disorder.

Treatment(s)
- Seek medical attention early
- Seek psychological counselling

# C

# CANCER

## Introduction

Cancer is a condition when abnormal tissues grow rapidly and can spread into surrounding tissues; usually referred to as malignant.

Cancer is a disease and it can be anywhere in your body. When diagnosed, it is a very personal matter. Many people still do not want to speak of cancer and behave as though it is a taboo subject.

Treatments include radiation, chemotherapy drugs (oral or intravenous), radium implants, hormonal therapy or surgery. There are many people who choose to use herbal medicine or nutritional therapy. We have had some friends who have chosen this route.

A cancer diagnosis demands early intervention. It is time to make the decision on your own or after speaking to family members.

Early detection, decision and intervention save lives. If there is a history of cancer in your family then you must be more in tune with your body and if you notice any changes, contact your doctor immediately.

A cancer diagnosis is a scary one, and often "Why Me?" is the first thought. A person with this diagnosis may go through periods of anger, frustration, depression, self-pity and isolation.

We both have many friends and family members with cancer, and we have supported and comforted them throughout their diagnosis, treatments, and care. Unfortunately, we have also lost many friends mainly from breast cancer.

Always remember that early diagnosis is key, and the support of family and friends is crucial during this emotional and unsettling period.

- Good eating habits:
    - Diet - watch what you eat closely, eat less fatty and processed foods
    - Drink lots of fluids
    - It is also important to incorporate servings of fruit and vegetables into every meal and snack

## CERVIX

### Introduction

The cervix is the lower portion of the uterus and opens into the vagina.

Cancer of the cervix is a problem with women. If it is discovered early the survival rate is very good. During your annual visit to your gynecologist a "Pap Smear" is taken, and when the test is completed the result is forwarded to your gynecologist or the physician who have ordered the test. If there are any abnormal findings, such as the presence of cancer cells there is a need for further tests and evaluations by your physician.

## CHEMOTHERAPY

### Introduction

Chemotherapy (also known as Chemo) treatments after a cancer diagnosis is a difficult time. Accepting that you have cancer is scary and to go through weeks of chemotherapy is tiring, and an added burden on you as well as your family.

The drug of choice, dosages and times for treatments are discussed with the oncologist (a doctor who specializes in cancer treatment). Once the decision is made chemotherapy may begin.

There are oral forms of chemotherapy as well as those that are administered through the veins.

Most women lose their hair during chemotherapy, and either wear a wig, turban, bandana, head scarf or remain bald. This is a very challenging time for a woman especially since her hair is a significant part of her sense of beauty and style.

During treatment, many women suffer from nausea and / or vomiting. Many successful strides have been made with the discovery of new drugs / therapies. However, Chemotherapy and / or Radiation remain the dominant options for treatment.


## CHILDBIRTH

<u>Introduction</u>

Childbirth is the end of pregnancy. (Please refer to the section on pregnancy)

What a relief for many of us, after nine long months of looking bloated, having swollen feet, strange food cravings and frequent bathroom visits. After carrying all this additional weight around it is time to get back to looking and feeling normal again! So, the labor pains start and how so many of us wish it can go as easy as some of our friends, in and out of the delivery room with speed. But alas, all of us have different experiences. Labor can last for a short or long period of time.

Oh well this must be taken in stride, but then after the baby is born, sit back and relax as everyone begins to 'coo' and spoil the infant.

A birth can be through a Cesarean section (Surgical procedures in the Operating room). There is an old saying that "once a C-section, always a C-section". This is no longer the case.

A new life begins! It is a happy time. A feeling of accomplishment, and the beginning of parenthood.

## CHLAMYDIA

Introduction

Chlamydia occurs when there is direct contact with infected mucus and secretions in the genitals, throat, and mouth.

Signs and Symptoms:
Many women have no Signs and Symptoms, but some do.
- A burning sensation when passing urine
- Abdominal pain (often times severe)
- Bleeding in between menstruation(periods)
- Pain during sex
- Vaginal discharge (minimal to a large amount)

Treatment(s)
- Antibiotics
- If Chlamydia is not treated you can develop a Pelvic Inflammatory Disease (PID) which can lead to infertility. You must be very careful, and if any of the above Signs and Symptoms are present when pregnant, the baby might develop an eye infection and / or pneumonia if untreated.

## CLITORIS

### Introduction

The clitoris is found in the inner lips of the vagina. It is a very sensitive organ that hardens with stimulation during sex and / or masturbation. This is also called the G-spot.

## COLON

### Introduction

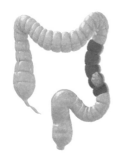

The colon is also called the large intestines, which is a part of the digestive system.

Food enters the mouth, goes into the stomach, and enters the bowels, which is also called the small intestines. From the bowels, the food travels to the rectum for excretion.

Stool is formed in the colon.

### Colon Conditions

- Colitis: Inflammation of the colon.
- Colon Bleeding (hemorrhage): Causes vary, and blood is often seen in the stool.
- Diverticulitis: This happens if or when diverticula becomes inflamed or infected. Some of the Signs and Symptoms are abdominal pain, fever, and constipation.
- Diverticulosis: Weak areas in the muscles of the colon which causes the colon's lining to protrude through the colon, forming tiny pouches called diverticuli. These usually cause no problems but can bleed or become inflamed or infected.

- Polyps: These are very small growths. They can develop and become cancerous. They are removed when discovered, for example, during colonoscopy; and sent to the laboratory to be evaluated.

## COLONOSCOPY

### Introduction

A colonoscopy is an internal examination of the colon (large intestine) and rectum. An instrument called a colonoscope is used to perform the procedure.

A baseline colonoscopy is recommended at age 45.

A colonoscopy is normally an outpatient procedure. You must have someone present to take you home because you will be drowsy from the sedative. You are cautioned not to drive after the procedure. Many outpatient areas will not perform this procedure if there is no one to take the patient home.

### Reasons for a Colonoscopy
A Colonoscopy may be done for the following reasons:
- A routine colonoscopy for the initial baseline, or follow up
- Abdominal pain
- Abnormal changes in polyps
- Abnormal weight loss
- Blood in the stool, or black, tarry stools
- Changes in bowel movements
- Inflammatory bowel disease
- Screening for colorectal cancer

## Preparation for a Colonoscopy

Your intestines must be properly emptied. You will be given instructions on how to do this, and these instructions must be specifically followed. If the colon is not clean or clear, the test would be cancelled. Tests preparation includes enemas, lots of fluid, food restriction and medication.

## Performing the Test

The colonoscope is attached to a small camera so that the entire colon can be seen.

You would be asked to lie on your side with your knees drawn up toward your chest. An anesthesiologist is usually present during the procedure and you will be given a mild sedative.

The gastroenterologist inserts the scope through the anus and moves it gently into the small intestine first. Air is inserted through the scope to provide a better view, and suction may be used to remove fluid or stool.

The colon is inspected very carefully and slowly so that the lining of the colon is not punctured and tissue samples are taken. Also as previously mentioned if there are any polyps present they will be removed and sent to the laboratory for testing.

## Results

- Abnormal - will be followed up by your doctor
- Normal - nothing else is required until next ordered colonoscopy

## COLPOSCOPY

### Introduction

A procedure used by your gynecologist for a pelvic exam to examine the vulva, vagina, and cervix closely. This procedure can help to detect cancer and any other possible findings.

## CHOLECYSTITIS (Acute)

### Introduction

Cholecystitis is swelling (inflammation) of the gall bladder. It is a potentially serious condition that usually needs to be treated in the hospital.

### Signs and Symptoms
- Bulging abdomen
- High temperature
- Jaundiced eyes
- Loss of appetite
- Nausea and vomiting
- Persistent pain that does not go away within a few hours
- Sudden sharp pain in the upper right side of your abdomen that spreads towards your right shoulder
- Sweating
- Tender abdomen
- Worsening pain with deep breaths
- Yellowing of the skin

### Causes
The main cause of Cholecystitis is when the main opening of the gall bladder is blocked by a gall stone. Bile builds up in the gall bladder and increases pressure inside which causes it to become inflamed.

There are other causes of Cholecystitis. This can be identified by your Primary Care Physician.

Diagnosis
- Abdominal examination
- Blood test to check for signs of inflammation
- Ultrasound of your abdomen to check for gall stones or other signs of a problem with your gall bladder

Treatment(s)
- Antibiotics
- Fasting
- Hospitalization, if necessary
- Increased fluid intake
- Pain medication
- Surgery, if necessary

Preventing Cholecystitis
- Eat a balanced diet
- Reduce fat intake
- Regular exercise
- Prevention is not always possible

## COUGH

Introduction

A cough is a reflex action which helps to keep the airway clear. Water or over the counter cough medications can help to reduce the cough. But if it persists for too long you must seek medical attention; especially if you smoke.

Remember, always cover your mouth when you cough, or cough in your shirt sleeves by bringing your bent arm to cover your mouth and nose. If people are present, turn your face away. This simple action stops the spread of germs and infections. Remember to wash your hands thoroughly afterwards.

If you have a persistent cough or you are coughing up blood you must seek medical attention immediately.

## CYSTOCELE

### Introduction

A cystocele occurs when the supportive tissue between a woman's bladder and vaginal wall weakens and stretches. This then allows the bladder to bulge into the vagina. A cystocele is also called a prolapsed bladder.

Straining the muscles that support the pelvic organs may lead to a cystocele. This can occur during a vaginal childbirth delivery, chronic constipation, violent coughing and lifting heavy items.

Surgery is not necessary if a cystocele does not present a problem. But, in some cases, surgery is necessary so that the vagina and other pelvic organs are not affected.

### Signs and Symptoms
In mild cases, there are no Signs and Symptoms.

Sometime later, Signs and Symptoms may occur, these are:
- A feeling that the bladder is not emptied after urinating
- Discomfort when straining, coughing, or lifting
- Feeling full or pressure in your pelvis and vagina when standing for long periods of time
- Recurrent bladder infections
- In severe cases, when the cystocele protrudes through the vaginal, the soft bulges are uncomfortable when sitting, but often goes away when lying down
- Pain or leaking urine during sexual intercourse

- Urine control is affected when laughing, sneezing or coughing. This can be very embarrassing. This is called stress incontinence

Most common causes
- A chronic cough
- Frequent straining of bowel movements
- Overweight or obese
- Pregnancy and vaginal childbirth (Women who have only cesarean section deliveries are less likely to develop prolapse)
- Repetitive heavy lifting

Performing Kegel exercises help to strengthen the pelvic floor muscles and also prevent and treat stress incontinence. To perform Kegel exercises, follow the following steps:
- Lie on your back with knees bent and feet placed on the floor, squeeze as though you are trying to stop urinating
- Hold this position for a count of three and then relax for a count of three
- Repeat 10 to 15 times
- Repeat 3 times daily

# CYSTS

## Introduction

Breast cysts: fluid-filled sacs that are tender during the menstrual cycle.

Ovarian cysts: Fluid-filled sacs.

# CYSTITIS

## Introduction

Cystitis is when there is severe stinging and pain during urination, along with the constant urge to pass urine. Cystitis is also known as a Urinary Tract Infection (UTI), and must be treated with the appropriate antibiotics. Also take the antibiotic and entire dosage recommended by your doctor. Do not reach for the one that is in your medicine cabinet.

Cystitis / UTI can also affect your sex life since intercourse may be painful during this time of infection.

*"I'm interested in women's health because I'm a woman. I'd be a darn fool not to be on my own side".*
Maya Angelou

# D

# DEPRESSION

## Introduction

Depression affects many women. It affects the mind and body, in both personal and work life. The old adage of calling depression "the blues" is taken more seriously now more than in the past.

Women also have mood changes due to hormonal reasons, such as during menstruation, menopause and pregnancy.

Women may develop depression after childbirth (postpartum depression), or after experiencing failed infertility treatments, miscarriages, and surgical procedures which cause early menopause.

It is observed that women are more likely than men to attempt suicide as a result of depression. However, men are more successful in their suicidal attempts than women. Every suicide threat should be taken seriously. It is extremely important to contact a mental health worker or medical professional immediately if someone you know makes a suicide threat. If you have suicidal thoughts, tell someone and seek help and / or counselling. See helpful contact information under references.

## Risk Factors

- Death of a parent, significant other, family members or friends
- Domestic violence
- Family history of mood disorders
- History of physical / sexual abuse
- Infertility
- Loss or threat of loss of social support system
- Personal history of mood disorders, particularly during the early reproductive years
- Rape
- Stress

Signs and Symptoms of Depression

- Changes in appetite including weight loss or weight gain
- Constant thoughts of death
- Depressed or irritable mood
- Difficulty concentrating or maintaining attention
- Feelings of guilt, hopelessness, and worthlessness
- General withdrawal
- Lack of energy or constant fatigue
- Loss / lack of interest in sex
- Not being able to sleep or sleeping too much (insomnia or hypersomnia)
- Recurrent suicidal thoughts
- Reduction of interest or pleasure in activities

## DIABETES

Introduction

Diabetes is a chronic disease which affects how your body turns food into energy. It is very common, and people over 45 years of age are more liable to get diabetes. Diabetes is caused when the blood glucose (known also as blood sugar is too high). This is caused when the body is not able to make enough insulin which is necessary to control blood sugar. Insulin is made by the pancreas and allows blood sugar into the cells for energy.

There are two types of diabetes:
Type 1
Type 2

## TYPE 1

This is when the body does not make any insulin. This affects children and younger people. Since their bodies cannot generate their own insulin, they must take manufactured insulin every day for the rest of their lives.

## TYPE 2

This can be developed at any age and is the most common type of diabetes. The body does not make or use insulin well. This occurs more often if there is a family history of diabetes.

## Gestational Diabetes

This is considered as a Type 2 Diabetes. It is developed only during pregnancy. Often pregnant women become concerned if they notice that their feet are more swollen than normal and seek medical attention, or this can be diagnosed during a routine pregnancy check up. Once the baby is born this often goes away.

## Signs and Symptoms
- Thirst
- Tiredness
- Weight Loss

## Prevention
- Diet
- Exercise
- Lose Weight

## Tests
- Blood Glucose (you must fast prior to this test)
- Urine Sample

Diabetes leads to other health problems such as:
- Dental problems
- Eye problems
- Foot problems
- Heart Disease
- Kidney Diseases
- Nerve damage
- Stroke
- Vascular / Circulatory problems

HYPERGLYCEMIA

(High blood sugar). Found in both Type 1 and Type 2 Diabetes.

Signs and Symptoms
- Blurred vision
- Cuts or sores that will not heal
- Excessive Thirst
- Fatigue
- Frequent urination
- Headaches
- Weight loss

Treatment(s)
- Annual eye exams
- Follow an exercise program
- If on medication, take as ordered
- Meet with a dietitian to determine dietary needs and prepare a diet plan
- See a podiatrist for help in foot care
- See endocrinologist (responsible for your treatment plan)
- Wear a medical identification for emergency purposes

## Self Care

A key thing to be aware of if you are a diabetic is not to cut or bruise yourself since open wounds are hard to heal. Many diabetics are referred to a podiatrist for assistance in keeping their toe nails trim.

Be sure to check your blood sugar every day and administer insulin daily as ordered.

## HYPOGLYCEMIA

(Low blood sugar). Most common in Type 1 Diabetes.

## Signs and Symptoms
- Confusion
- Disorientation
- Dizziness
- Headaches
- Hunger
- Paleness
- Palpitations
- Seizure
- Sweating
- Unconsciousness

## Treatments:
- Avoid wearing tight shoes or socks
- Daily Glucose testing either by finger stick or one of the other modern methods
- Eat meals on time
- Glucose tablets
- High sugar foods and drinks
- If on insulin, have a meal before administering insulin
- Monitor for poor circulation especially in your extremities (hands and feet)

- No smoking
- Only drink small / moderate amount of alcohol
- Orange juice, soda, candy
- Take medications as prescribed

Self Care
- Some diabetics monitor themselves very well, they are keenly aware of the signs of low blood sugar and immediately drink some orange juice or eat a candy

## PRE-DIABETES

Introduction

The blood sugar is higher than normal, but not enough to be diagnosed as diabetes. You can cut your risk of developing diabetes which is usually Type 2 by changing your lifestyle. Change your diet, start and maintain an exercise routine, lose weight, seek the assistance of a nutritionist. I know many people who are pre-diabetic and have done all of the above and have lost significant weight in managing their condition.

Recently I (Sylvia) was traveling with a friend who offered me a snack which she thought was a healthy one. It had pecans, maple, glazed mix walnuts, apples, cherries and cinnamon. She said it was "yummy" and asked me to try it. I did, and immediately told her that I do not use sugar and the items were too sweet.

Out of the blue she said, 'I guess it's 'Diabetes in a Bag.' I told her she has just coined a new term and incidentally I was writing about Diabetes in this book at the time.

# DIET

## Introduction

A healthy diet consists of drinking lots of water and eating vegetables, proteins, multi grains, and fruits. It is as simple as that. Eat in moderation and when hungry. Eat small portions, avoid greasy and fatty foods. Please refer to the Food Pyramid which is the U.S. Department of Agriculture's updated guide to better nutrition.

 In some cultures the first drink in the morning is a cup of hot water, you can add lemon if you choose to do so. Try not to eat late in the evening. We recommend that you do not eat after 8 pm. And remember to chew your food properly. We know many friends who are now drinking a glass of water before each meal because they feel the water fills them sufficiently and they tend not to overeat.

Also add healthy foods to your diet, at least five to seven servings of food high in antioxidants. Foods such as:
- Broccoli
- Kidney beans
- Tomatoes (not canned)

Your diet should also include foods high in Omega 3 Fats. Such as:
- Fish
- Flaxseed
- Soybean
- Squash
- Walnuts

Foods high in fiber are:
- Beans
- Flax meal
- Lentils
- Peas

Foods you should avoid are:
- Enriched Flour
- High Fructose corn syrup
- Saturated Fats- animal fats
- Sugar
- Trans fat - Hydrogenated Oils

A well-balanced diet helps you to keep your weight down, keep you healthy, and make you feel and look good.

*Hint: Read the ingredient list when grocery shopping. Check the contents for sugar, added sugar, salt, protein, fat etc. If you cannot pronounce it, do not eat it!*

DOUCHING

Introduction

Douching is a method that is used to wash out the vagina, usually with a mixture of water and vinegar. However, some douches also contain antiseptics and fragrances. Most women who douche buy a commercial preparation sold in drugstores and supermarkets.

A small percentage of women use a homemade mixture of water and vinegar or water alone. A Douche application comes in a bottle or bag and is sprayed upward into the vagina through a tube. Some women say douching makes them feel cleaner.

However, be cautious, douching is not recommended because it washes away good bacteria, and can push infection up into the fallopian tubes, especially after sex.

*"Women's health needs to be front, and center-it often isn't, but it needs to be."*
Cynthia Nixon

# E

# ECTOPIC PREGNANCY

Introduction

This occurs when an egg (ova) is fertilized and grows outside of the womb. When this happens the fertilized egg / ova does not develop into a baby.

A pregnant woman usually does not know that something is wrong, and will continue to enjoy her pregnancy until she has a routine visit to her doctor or something goes wrong that makes a gynecologist's visit necessary, for example, abdominal pain and / or vaginal bleeding.

If there are any signs and symptoms, this usually starts around week 5 to 12 of the pregnancy.

Some Signs and Symptoms are:
- Abdominal pain, typically only on one side that can range from mild to severe
- Abnormal vaginal bleeding

Treatment(s):
- Medication in the early stage to stop the fertilized egg (ova) from growing
- Surgery will be necessary. If left untreated the fallopian tube can rupture. If it does, this will be an emergency situation
- The fertilized egg (ova) may die on its own

Some signs of fallopian tube rupture are:
- Diarrhea
- Feeling faint and dizzy
- Sudden onset of severe pain

Some things that increase the risk of ectopic pregnancy include:

- A previous history of ectopic pregnancy (ies)
- Pelvic Inflammatory Disease (PID)
- Smoking

Losing a baby can be devastating and women go through a grieving process. But, you can try for another baby after discussion with your gynecologist. In the past women died from having an ectopic pregnancy. But, these days, with early diagnosis and treatment, death is preventable.

## ECZEMA

### Introduction

Eczema is a general term for any type of dermatitis or "itchy rash". There are several skin diseases that are eczemas and they all cause itching and redness. Some will blister, weep or peel. Please do not scratch. Scratching will open the blisters which can become infected and delay healing.

### Treatment(s)
- Medication (Over-the-counter (OTC) )
- See a dermatologist

# ENDOMETRIOSIS

## Introduction

Endometriosis occurs when clumps of the uterine lining grow outside the uterus. Severe cases may make it necessary for a hysterectomy (surgical procedure) to be performed. Endometritis may also cause infertility.

## Signs and Symptoms
- Abdominal tenderness
- Heavy bleeding during menstruation
- Pain with bowel movement and / or urination
- Painful intercourse
- Severe menstrual cramps

## Diagnosis
- Pelvic exam
- Ultrasound

## Treatment
- Hormone medication
- Pain medication
- Self care
- Surgery, if indicated

# ENDOMETRITIS

## Introduction

Endometritis is the inflammation or irritation of the endometrium, which is the mucus membrane lining the uterus.

## Signs and Symptoms
- Abdominal pain
- Discomfort during bowel movement
- Fever
- Painful periods
- Vaginal bleeding or discharge

## Diagnosis
- Colposcopy
- Pap smear

## Treatment
- Antibiotics as prescribed by your physician
- Anti inflammatory drugs as prescribed by your physician

Your sexual partner needs to be informed of your diagnosis.

# ENERGY/ EXERCISE

## Introduction

At times, a woman is both mother and father to her child (children) and needs her energy to handle the day to day requirements of being a parent. This also relates to non-parent, single women.

It is important to add daily exercise to your daily routine, making sure to take the time to do this. It will help to relieve stress and to promote health. Healthy eating is also a vital part of self maintenance for parents.

Our children depend on us to be available and we cannot be there for them unless we are well.

There are Metabolism Boosters that can be used to help increase your metabolism in order to burn fat. Such as:

- Beans - red, white and black
- Oolong Tea
- Spicy tomato juice

Before you begin any exercise routine you MUST first check with your doctor. It is also best to have an exercise buddy because he/she can encourage you when you do not feel like exercising.

Start slow, take deep breaths and MOVE!

START- Start from somewhere, anywhere - just start to MOVE!

# F

# FALLOPIAN TUBES

## Introduction

There are two Fallopian tubes also known as the uterine tubes, one on each side of the uterus. These tubes are part of the female reproductive system and allow for the eggs to pass from the ovaries to the uterus.

# FIBROADENOMA

## Introduction

Fibroadenoma are lumps that are painless and move around in the breast tissue. They are caused by an excess of milk-producing glands and is found in women between the ages of 20 to 30 years old. A new lump or change in the breast must be evaluated by a doctor.

# FIBROCYSTIC BREASTS

## Introduction

These are lumps in the breast that are non- cancerous. The breast may feel dense, tender, swollen and painful under the armpit. The lumps are caused by changes in hormone balance and may show up before the menstrual period. This usually affect women between the ages of 35 to 50 years.

If you are diagnosed with fibrocystic breasts, it is very important to be closely monitored by your physician and you MUST have your annual mammogram, and some professionals may recommend ultrasound.

Fibrocystic breasts do not usually increase your risk of breast cancer.

Treatment(s):
- Breast biopsy if recommended by your doctor
- Monitor for changes in the feel and size of the breast
- Surgery if recommended by your doctor

## FIBROIDS

### Introduction

A fibroid is made up mostly of muscle tissue. It can be as small as a pea or as big as an orange, grapefruit or cantaloupe. Fibroids are usually non-cancerous and can develop at any age.

A fibroid is one of the things that we can certainly live without, and for unknown reasons are mostly prevalent in black women.

The cause of fibroids is not well understood. The risk factors include family history, obesity, early puberty and stress.

### Signs and Symptoms
- Heavy monthly periods and consequent blood loss can sometimes lead to serious anemia, weakness and cramping
- Fibroids sometimes shrink as you reach menopause. For younger women fibroids need to be monitored to see how they grow, and how quickly they grow
- Some women are not aware that they have fibroids, but others experience heavy bleeding, cramping, abdominal pressure, swelling of the abdomen, frequent urination, painful intercourse, fatigue, miscarriages and infertility
- It might be necessary to surgically remove the fibroids

Treatment(s)
- Birth control
- Embolization is a less invasive procedure, to shrink uterine fibroids by blocking off their blood supply
- Hormone therapy
- Hysterectomy (the removal of the uterus). This can be partial or total. We have seen women who have opted for the Myomectomy and later have had to eventually have a Hysterectomy since fibroids can reoccur
- Insertion of an IUD (Intrauterine device)
- Myomectomy (the removal of the fibroid only)

Alternative Treatment(s) for Fibroids
- Drink caffeine in moderation
- Eat fish rich in Omega 3 (salmon or sardines)
- Eat more fruits and vegetables and less meat
- Exercise
- Limit weekly wine intake, no more than 5 glasses per week

# G

# GENITAL WARTS

## Introduction

Genital warts, like herpes is a contagious Sexually Transmitted Disease (STD). It is also spread through sexual contact during sex by someone who is already infected.

## Signs and Symptoms
- Bleeding (Occasionally)
- Discharge
- Itching
- Painless red bumps
- Ulcers
- Urinary Obstruction

## Treatment(s)
- Apply medication directly to the warts
- Avoid unprotected sex (use a condom)
- Can be surgically removed
- Do not pick at the warts
- Tell your sexual partner
- Your medical caregiver will instruct you regarding the best mode of treatment

# GONORRHEA

## Introduction

Gonorrhea ( is also known as CLAP) It is a Sexually Transmitted Disease (STD), and is one of the most common.

One can have a repeat if he / she has sex again with an infected partner. If gonorrhea is left untreated Pelvic Inflammatory Disease (PID) and infertility may occur (Please see later section).

To avoid an STD you can do so either by abstinence or having the person wear a protective device (condom). It is the woman's responsibility to protect herself.

## Transmission

Direct contact from your sexual partner through the vagina, anus, mouth or penis.

## Signs and Symptoms
- Abnormal discharge from the vagina which can be watery, creamy or light green
- Burning, painful urination
- Develop within 2-10 days after having sex with an infected person
- Fever, pus, sore throat and the frequent urge to urinate
- Mild to no symptoms in women
- Pain during sexual intercourse

## Treatment(s)
- Antibiotics, as prescribed by your physician

# GRAVE'S DISEASE

## Introduction

Grave's disease is an immune system disorder caused by an overactive thyroid which means the immune system mistakes something in the body as being toxic and attacks the thyroid glands. Because of this the thyroid produces excessive hormones which causes Grave's disease.

It is most common in women aged 20 to 40 years old and can run in families. You are more likely to develop this disease if you smoke.

People with Grave's disease usually have abnormally large or puffy eyes.

## Signs and Symptoms

- Bulging / Puffy eyes
- Hair loss
- Hand tremors
- Heat sensitivity
- High blood pressure
- Large thyroid
- Weight loss

## Treatment(s)

- Anti-thyroid medication
- Radiation therapy
- Radioactive iodine
- Surgery to remove the thyroid

Graves' disease may run in families. Examinations of the members of a family may reveal other individuals with this disease.

# GYNECOLOGIST

## Introduction

A gynecologist is a doctor who deals mainly with females. This is one of the doctors you must be sure to see annually for your pap smear / pap test, breast and pelvic examinations. The gynecologist also checks the laboratory work for women who are close to menopause. This check is to determine hormonal levels and subsequent discussions as necessary.

The earliest age for you to see a gynecologist is either when the menstrual periods begin or if there is any other conditions that warrants a visit. In some young women the menstruation periods begin earlier than others.

Some women prefer a female gynecologist to care for her. Here again, you are making a personal decision.

*"Communities and countries and ultimately the world are only as strong as the health of their women."*
Michelle Obama

# HEART

## Introduction

The normal heart is said to be the size of one's clenched fist. It is

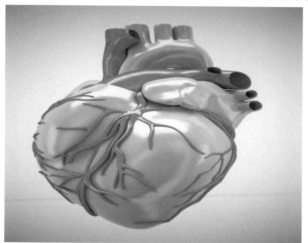

found on the left side of the chest. It pumps blood through the arteries and veins. The arteries, veins and heart is called the cardiovascular system.

The heart has four chambers, two right and two left. These are responsible for receiving blood, making sure there is enough oxygen; and pumps the blood filled with oxygen to the lungs and other organs of the body. This is called the circulatory system.

The normal heart rate of an adult is between 80 to 100 beats per minute. For an athletic person, the heart rate can be as low as 40 beats per minute.

If there is an existence of a low heart rate and the following signs and symptoms are present, such as shortness of breath, dizziness, fainting, sweating. Call your physician and / or your emergency number; and go to the nearest Emergency Department.

# HEART ATTACK

## Introduction

A heart attack is also called a Myocardial Infarction (MI). A heart attack is caused by a build up of plaque(fat) in the arteries. The arteries are vessels in the heart that carries nutrients and oxygen during circulation. When there is a build up of plaque, blood cannot get to the heart muscle and it dies which causes a heart attack.

## Signs and Symptoms

- Anxiety
- Chest pain which radiates to the left arm
- Difficulty in breathing
- Dizziness
- Indigestion
- Nausea or vomiting
- Pain in the left upper jaw
- Sweating
- Unusual fatigue

In women the signs and symptoms of a heart attack are most often different than in men. We have little or no pain on the left side. There might be a cold sweat, or complaint of an upset stomach or pain in the abdomen, shortness of breath, nausea or back pain.

It is documented that women have signs and symptoms of a heart attack weeks or months before diagnosis. Women suffer what is called a "silent heart attack" and more women than men go undiagnosed when there is a heart condition.

Among the leading cause of death in women, a heart attack is number one. If the pain persists or there is a family history of heart disease you MUST seek medical help immediately. If you suspect a heart attack call 911 or the emergency number in the state in which you reside.

**The brain can only live up to 4 minutes without oxygen.**

There are many places where you can take a Basic Cardiac Life Support (BCLS) or a Cardiopulmonary Resuscitation (CPR) class that teaches you emergency measures. Check your local Red Cross or Health Department for sites and availability.

## HEMORRHOIDS

Introduction

Hemorrhoids are also known as Piles. They are swollen and inflamed veins in the lower end of the anus (rectum) and can be either internal (just inside the anus) or external (at the anal opening). This can protrude and hang outside the anus (rectum). Hemorrhoids in women often occur during pregnancy.

Many women are embarrassed to admit that they have hemorrhoids. You should not be!

Signs and Symptoms
- Blood in the stool
- Itching at the anal area
- Pain when having a bowel movement
- Pain when seated

Causes
- Anal infections
- Constipation
- Obesity
- Pregnancy
- Straining during bowel movements

Diagnosis
- Digital examination
- Rectal examination
- Sigmoidoscopy is an internal examination of the lower large bowel and rectum. An instrument called a sigmoidoscope is used. This has a light attached to it providing the doctor's with a clearer view of the anus. This procedure can be done in the Primary Care doctor's office.

Treatment(s)
- Avoid scented toilet tissue
- Do not scratch the area (your fingernails can cause bleeding and introduce infection)
- Drink plenty water
- Eat a diet high in fiber, for example oats, beans, apples, flax seeds
- Sitz baths, which is a warm soothing soak for your bottom area, are also options
- Stool softener
- Surgical removal
- Wear cotton panties

## HERPES

Introduction

There are two types of Herpes, Genital Herpes (Herpes Type 2 and Oral Herpes (Herpes Type 1). Both are caused by the herpes simplex virus (HSV).

Genital herpes is a Sexually Transmitted Disease (STD). It is transmitted by unprotected sex through the vagina, or by oral and anal sex. Contrary to common thought, you cannot get genital herpes by sitting on a dirty toilet seat or chair.

Genital herpes can go undetected for years. But, if you have pain, itching, sores on the penis, vagina or the buttocks; it is best to seek medical advice. Do not scratch. If you have a sexual partner you must let the person know as soon as you are sure, so that he / she can seek medical care.

Oral Herpes looks like fever blisters on the lips and around the mouth and is transmitted by kissing someone who has herpes.

There is no cure for herpes, but it can go into remission. Be aware that during remission you may unknowingly transmit the virus.

Symptoms (Genital)
There may not be any symptoms that are visible, but the following can be present.
- Burning upon urination / Having trouble passing urine
- Itching, pain around the genitals
- Fever and chills
- Swollen glands

Symptoms (Oral)
- Cold sores or fever blisters, sores on lips, around the mouth
- Sores inside the mouth

Treatment(s)
- Avoid kissing someone who has oral herpes
- Avoid unprotected sex until the disease is cured
- Keep sores as clean as possible
- Take pain medication

HOT FLASHES—PRIVATE SUMMERS

Introduction

Hot flashes are sometimes referred to as 'private summers.' These occur during menopause. This is an uncomfortable and annoying period for many women. But, some fortunate women do not have this experience.

We have seen many of our friends and colleagues when they get a hot flash, they begin to fan themselves with anything at hand, frustrated as they wish this agony will go away.   Many women wake during the night drenched in sweat, and either have to change their clothing or take a shower to cool down.

Is there a treatment or cure for this?   How do you put the fire out? There are many ideas that work for some, but not for others. There are a few over the counter remedies such as:
- Black Cohosh
- Dandelion Tea
- Evening Primrose oil
- Soy Isoflavones
- Vitamin E

Your gynecologists or Primary Care Physician will have other recommendations for you.


## HYSTERECTOMY

### Introduction

A Hysterectomy is the removal of the uterus, and occasionally the ovaries.   A partial hysterectomy is when there is only the removal of the uterus. A total hysterectomy is when the uterus, fallopian tubes, ovaries and cervix are removed. A hysterectomy can be performed through the vagina or by abdominal incision. Robotic surgery is now an option.

### Signs and Symptoms
- Cancer
- Endometritis
- Enlarged fibroids
- Heavy and prolonged blood loss during menstrual periods

- Prolapsed uterus

Treatment(s) /Surgical Procedure

At the present time, a hysterectomy is no longer the lengthy procedure compared to past years. It can be done by laparoscopic surgery which is not as invasive; the woman is left with very small incisions, and the recovery time is much less. This enables the woman to return to her day to day activities sooner and many women can still wear their swimsuits and bikinis because of the smaller scars.

There is much controversy as to when a hysterectomy is necessary. Again, this is a woman's personal choice. It is more indicated for excessive bleeding or if a fibroid is growing so rapidly that they might actually be tumors. It should not be the first option.

Many women hesitate to have a hysterectomy based on the old adage that a woman is not complete if the uterus is removed. It is an easier decision to make once a woman has had children. However, this can be a very emotional, and often traumatic decision for a woman who is contemplating pregnancy.

An active sex life can continue after a hysterectomy, but having a hysterectomy can also cause a loss of fertility, and for some women, sexual dysfunction.

I

# ITCHING

## Introduction

Itching is an irritating sensation and scratching the area is a natural reaction to relieve this discomfort.

Any form of prolonged itching with discharge in the vaginal area must be addressed since it can be a sign of infection. Any infection must be treated with the appropriate antibiotics.

Remember, never treat yourself at any time with antibiotics that was left over from a previous prescription. Each infection is different and should be diagnosed by a doctor, who will prescribe the appropriate treatment.

## Treatment(s)

- Apply topical anesthesia, if indicated
- Avoid scratching
- Have oatmeal baths
- Keep skin clean
- Moisturize dry skin
- See a dermatologist when necessary

# J

# JOINT DISEASES

## Introduction

Joint disease is any disease that affects the joints, such as arthritis which is the most common. We have discussed some of these conditions in previous sections of this book.

Pain in any joint which causes discomfort and the inability to move the pain affected area freely.

# K

# KIDNEYS

## Introduction

The kidneys are a pair of organs located in the back of the abdomen. Each kidney is about 4 or 5 inches long - about the size of a fist.

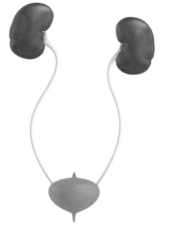

The kidneys' functions are to filter blood, remove waste, control the body's fluid balance, and regulate the balance of electrolytes (salt, potassium, calcium etc.). The kidneys filter blood which create urine. The urine collects in the kidneys and drain down through tubes called ureters to the bladder.

If the kidneys stop working it is necessary to go on dialysis to remove waste from the body. If a family member is on dialysis and needs a kidney transplant any family member, or friends can be tested. If he/she is a match a kidney transplant can be performed.

A person can live a full life with one kidney, so do not be afraid to donate. The doctor who treats a patient with a kidney disease must be a renal specialist, and will discuss all details with you before the transplant is performed.

There are many outreach efforts in place for organ donation and you can call and register as an organ donor. You do not have to wait until a family or friend is in need since there are numerous people waiting for a transplant of any organ.

Anyone can register to be a kidney donor at anytime or this can be done when you renew your driver's license. Your family should be informed that you are a registered organ donor.

Some common types of kidney diseases are:
- Kidney Stones
- Urinary Track Infection (UTI)

Signs and Symptoms
- Abdominal pain (severe, sharp and sudden)
- Back pain
- Blood in the urine
- Change in urination
- Frequent urination
- Nausea
- Sweating
- Vomiting

Treatment(s)
- Kidney Stones – see the doctor, drink lots of fluids. Stones may pass naturally or be surgically removed
- Urinary Track Infections (UTIs) - Antibiotics

*"Above all. Be the heroine of your life, not the victim."*

Nora Ephron

L

# LUMPS (Breast)

## Introduction

When a breast lump is detected it is best to seek medical help immediately. Women have been known to hide the fact that they have a breast lump, and have waited too long to seek medical advice.

We know friends who waited too long to seek medical advice and the outcome was that it was too late. By the time they decided to act, the cancer had spread to other vital organs and they died.

In our opinion, you should not be too engrossed in your body image in the fear of most likely having a mastectomy. The priority here should be to maintain your health in an attempt to prolong life.

Often, even with cancers that have spread, there have been cases when surgery, followed by chemotherapy and / or radiation, has helped to prolong life.

## Diagnosis
Diagnosis for a lump will be biopsy and ultrasound.

## Treatment(s)
Treatment will be based on diagnostic findings.


# LUPUS (Systemic Lupus Erythematosus)

## Introduction

Lupus is a chronic, autoimmune disease that can affect the skin, joints, kidneys, brain, heart, lungs and blood cells.  Chronic means that the signs and symptoms tend to last longer than six weeks and often for many years.

In lupus, the immune system breaks down and is unable to recognize the difference between viruses and healthy tissues; and creates its own antibodies that attack and destroy the healthy tissue.

These antibodies cause inflammation, pain, and damage in various parts of the body.

Lupus is an unpredictable disease. It flares up, the signs and symptoms may worsen, and you may feel ill. Then, it may go into remission, as the signs and symptoms improve, and you may feel better.

Lupus can range from mild to life-threatening and should always be treated by a doctor most often a rheumatologist. With good medical care, people with lupus can lead a full life. We have a friend who is still alive although she was diagnosed over thirty years ago.

Lupus is not contagious and affects mostly women of child bearing age, but anyone can develop this disease.

People of all races and ethnicity can develop lupus, but women of color are 2 to 3 times more likely to develop the disease.

Signs and Symptoms
The signs and symptoms are like many other illness and diseases.
- Chest pain
- Dry eyes
- Dry mouth
- Hair loss
- Joint pain
- Mouth ulcers
- Recurrent fever spells
- Skin rash

<u>Diagnosis</u>
- Current Signs and Symptoms
- Laboratory test results
- Medical history (including family members)
- Repeat lab test if necessary. A test result may be positive at one time and negative at another time
- Use same laboratory. Different laboratories may produce different test results

<u>Treatment(s)</u>
Discuss treatment options with your doctor.
- Diet and lifestyle changes
- Medications are important for managing many systemic lupus erythematosus (SLE) patients
- Numerous drug therapies are now available, and have assisted in better results than previously
- Self care (use sun block)

# M

# MASTECTOMY

Please review the section labelled 'Breast Cancer.'

## Introduction

The removal of a breast is a traumatic and emotional experience. Many women pride themselves in having large, well-rounded breasts, and often joke about flat-chested women.

When it becomes necessary to remove a breast the cosmetic issue is a difficult one. The decision for a mastectomy is one that is made with a lot of soul-searching.

Once the decision is made to have the breast removed, it is best to obtain the services of a surgeon who specializes in breast surgery.

After the surgery you will have a simple drain at the operative site to remove any excess fluid, and there will be swelling and pain. Speak to your healthcare provider about managing your pain since pain management aids your comfort and assists in an easier post-op recovery. Currently, to prepare the breast for reconstruction a decision may be made to insert an expander during surgery.

After a mastectomy, emotional support is needed from family and friends. There are also many support groups available in most communities and it is recommended that you join one. A strong suggestion is for your caregiver or partner to attend support group meetings with you. Studies show that black women develop breast cancer earlier than any other race.

# MENOPAUSE

## Introduction

Oh, the dreaded time of our lives! The periods stop. And although each month we have complained or cried in agony because of abdominal cramps; when the periods finally stop it causes an emotional upheaval.

Menopause --- the beginning of a new 'period'. Listen up, we cannot avoid aging, it is a fact of life.

Treatment(s) for menopause is a personal decision. Whether the choice is for a Hormone Replacement Therapy (HRT), herbal remedy, or nothing at all. See the 'Hot Flashes' section.

While more women will have a level of hormonal and emotional upheaval during menopause, other women are fortunate to go silently into the sunset of their womanhood! You can also experience signs and symptoms of early menopause after a hysterectomy.

# MENSTURATION / MENSTRUAL CYCLE

## Introduction

Menstruation (called a 'period') is the shedding and bleeding of the uterine lining. It is a normal occurrence in reproductive-age females. Blood flows from the uterus (womb) through the vagina. Regular menstruation lasts between 3 to 5 days.

Menorrhagia, a longer period is due to hormonal problems / uterine cancer.

Amenorrhea is the absence or menstrual periods caused by natural hormonal changes and does not necessarily mean that there is a problem.

The menstrual cycle sometimes is very annoying to many women because it interrupts their lifestyle. Although with some women it is business as usual. Many feel that they cannot have or enjoy intercourse during this time because it is too messy.

Some women elect to have 3 to 4 cycles per year for various reasons, such as a stop for vacation or other important events. They visit their healthcare professional and are placed on hormonal treatments or birth control pills. Newer treatment(s) may offer even less cycles per year.


## MITTELSCHMERZ (The Pain between Periods)

### Introduction

Mittelschmertz is pelvic pain that occurs between menstrual cycles during ovulation; hence the name Mittelschmerz, which comes from the German words for "middle" and "pain."

The pain usually occurs in the lower abdomen and pelvis either in the middle or to one side. It can range from a mild twinge to severe discomfort, lasting from minutes to hours. In some cases a small amount of vaginal bleeding or discharge might occur.

### Causes

As an egg develops in the ovary, it is surrounded by follicular fluid. During ovulation, the egg and the fluid, as well as some blood, are released from the ovary. While the exact cause of Mittelschmerz is unknown, it is believed that the fluid or blood might irritate the lining of the abdominal cavity causing pain. The pain goes away once the body absorbs the fluid or blood.

Signs and Symptoms

- Fever
- Mid-cycle pain lasting longer than a day
- Nausea
- Pain with urination
- Severe lower abdominal pain
- Vomiting

Diagnosis

Ovulation usually occurs about two weeks after the first day of each menstrual cycle, so the timing of the pain makes Mittelschmerz easy to recognize. To help determine if your pain is related to ovulation, your doctor might ask you to chart your menstrual cycles, noting any episodes of pain, as well as the location of the pain.

In addition, your doctor may perform an abdominal and pelvic examination to rule out other possible causes of pain, such as endometriosis or an ovarian cyst. If your pain is severe or if the doctor notices any irregularities on the exam, he or she may order blood tests or X-rays / ultrasound to determine the cause of your pain.

Treatment(s)

The pain usually goes away within about 24 hours, so specific treatment is not required. Over-the-counter pain medicines—such as ibuprofen—generally are effective in relieving Mittelschmerz. Women with particularly painful ovulation might find relief by taking birth control pills, which prevent ovulation.

Prevention

Preventing ovulation, which can be done with birth control pills, is the only way to effectively prevent Mittelschmerz.

# MISCARRIAGE

## Introduction

A miscarriage is the spontaneous loss of a fetus before the 20th week of pregnancy. (Pregnancy losses after the 20th week are called preterm deliveries.)

A miscarriage may also be called a "spontaneous abortion." This refers to naturally occurring events.

Other terms for the early loss of pregnancy include:
- Complete abortion: All of the products of conception leave the body
- Incomplete abortion: Only some of the products of conception leave the body
- Inevitable abortion: The signs and symptoms of abortion cannot be stopped, and a miscarriage occurs
- Infected abortion: when the lining of the womb, or uterus and any remaining products of conception become infected during an induced abortion; or by the use of dirty instruments or poor aseptic techniques
- Missed abortion: a miscarriage in which the fetus was not formed or has died in the womb. The fetus must be removed by the obstetrician

## Causes, incidence, and risk factors
Most miscarriages are caused by chromosome problems that make it impossible for the baby to develop. Usually, these problems are unrelated to the mother or father's genes.

Other possible causes for miscarriage include:
- Age of mother
- Hormone problems
- Incompetent cervix (a medical term – when the cervix opens too early during pregnancy)

- Infection
- Physical problems with the mother's reproductive organs
- Problem with the body's immune response
- Serious diseases in the mother (such as uncontrolled diabetes)

Signs
- Bleeding
- Fatigue
- Lack of movements of the fetus / baby
- Leakage of fluid from the vagina
- Nausea
- Pain (Abdominal, lower back and pelvic)
- Spotting
- Vomiting

Prevention
- Avoid alcohol and illegal drugs
- Eat healthy meals
- Exercises
- Maintain a healthy weight
- Manage stress
- A Shirodkar stitch is a sort of purse string stich put into the cervix to keep it tightly closed during pregnancy. This procedure helps to prevent a miscarriage)

# MOTHERHOOD

## Introduction

What a glorious time in a woman's life. You are finally a mother! You can nurture and give your child/children all that is good. Many women choose this time to relive the past and hope for the future. The things that you did not have, you are now going to make sure that they are available for your child / children.

Mothers often say that they make sacrifices for their child / children, but we disagree. When you become a mother what you give to your child / children, is given with love. Show and lead by example, remember you are preparing this child / children for the next stages of life. You want your child / children to succeed, to be the best they can be.

Whether or not you are a single parent your child / children should be your priority. We are proud parents. Betty has a daughter, Krystal; and I have a son, Josyl.

Mother's Day 2010 fell on my birthday and I received the following note from my son. It is with his permission that I insert it into this book.

May 8, 2010

Mom,

I thought this would be far more appropriate than another birthday or Mother's Day card, mostly because you share in all that I do and accomplish. Although I do my best to be a man of his own drive, I hope you realize that I only do so because I want to want for nothing just so that you can be comfortable in not wanting for me. I am happy and grateful to share my most recent victory with you because I never would have made it without you. As hard as I have worked, and as many hours and days, as I spent working to make a way for myself to lighten your load in taking on my burdens, I still would not have made it without you. I hope you know that I am never ignorant of that and that all your efforts and sacrifices provide my main motivation each day.

It is for this reason, among literally thousands, that I don't want to just say Happy Birthday anymore and don't want to just say Happy Mother's Day. I really want to say thank you eternally for all that you have done, all that you did not need to do, and all that you could not help yourself from doing for me. It helps me to go forward in the knowledge that, no matter what, I will always have you to lean on when I don't have the means to make it on my own. It also makes me keep going forward, no matter what the odds, knowing that you have blazed your trail in front of me, but would still always be there at my back at the same time. Such a love is truly astonishing to me, and it makes me yearn to have my own children just so I can know the gratification of showing that sort of unconditional love upon another. I do in fact feel selfish in keeping it for my own.

All of that being said, I truly just want to say thank you again. I wish I could say it many times each day. You have been an amazing matriarch to me, our family as it is, and the family that will come long after you and I are both gone from this Earth. Your spirit of giving, as God's trust vessel of love, is so powerful that it captivates all while paralyzing at the same time. This is something that you should be eternally proud of. More than anything my wish is to continue in the same spirit and make you proud with all that I am able to accomplish, in order to repay you for always creating the means and paving the way.

With love, many thanks, and great wishes for a Happy Birthday,

Your Son!

# MYOMECTOMY

## Introduction

A myomectomy is a procedure to surgically remove uterine fibroids from the uterus, but leave healthy tissues in case the woman wants to get pregnant later. Some women choose to do this instead of having a hysterectomy. Women who are past childbearing age or who do not want children might choose to have a hysterectomy instead since fibroids can recur after a myomectomy.

This is a personal decision.

# N

# NIGHT SWEATS

## Introduction

Night sweats can be normal. It can be caused by sleeping with your bedroom too hot or with too many covers. Other causes can be pre menopause changes, and / or decrease / increase in hormones, thyroid problems, and / or elevated cholesterol. It can also be caused by anxiety, the side effects of medication, and the inability of the hypothalamus gland which regulates body temperature.

If you have always suffered from night sweats and there is no medical reason, continue to monitor yourself. Any sudden or worrisome increase should be discussed with your doctor.

# NUTRITION

## Introduction

Remember the old adage "an apple a day keeps the doctor away." Eat well, plenty fruits, vegetables, and remember to drink lots and lots of water.

If you do not like plain water, add flavor, such as lemon or lime juices. Still, have a problem with water? Another solution can be another juice such as apple and cranberry etc.

OK, OK, just drink something. Drink something! And preferably try for at least eight glasses of fluid daily.

# OBESITY

## Introduction

Obesity is a disorder of excess body fat. Obesity is measured by the body mass index (BMI). A woman is considered overweight with a BMI between 25 and 29.9; and considered obese with a BMI over 30. Morbid obesity is a BMI of 40 or higher. Being overweight interferes with your overall health.

Your BMI can be calculated by your physician, nutritionist or yourself (use an internet search engine to find a BMI formula).

## Causes

Consistently consuming more calories than the body can burn causes obesity. For many people, this boils down to eating too much and exercising too little. But there are other factors that also play a role in becoming obese, such as:

- Age: As you get older, your body's ability to break down food slows down and you do not require as many calories to maintain your weight. It is extremely important to watch what you eat and continue to exercise. And, during menopause you should carefully monitor your food intake

- Environmental factors: Such as not having access healthy foods
- Gender: Women tend to be more overweight than men
- Genetics: Obesity tends to run in families
- Illness: Some illnesses can cause obesity. These include hormone problems such as hypothyroidism, where the thyroid is functioning poorly; depression and hormone treatments
- Medication: Certain drugs, such as steroids and some antidepressants, may cause excessive weight gain
- Physical activity: Individuals who are very active, should eat to maintain their weight. Additionally, physical activity

tends to decrease appetite in obese individuals while increasing the body's ability to metabolize fat as an energy source
- Psychological factors: Psychological factors also influence eating habits and obesity. Many people eat in response to emotions such as boredom, sadness, or anger. Some people cannot control how much they eat and how often

Treatment(s)
Depending on the causes, treatment can include the following:
- Diet
- Exercise
- Hydration
- Medical prescription / monitoring / management
- Weight loss
- Weight loss surgery


OSTEOPOROSIS

Introduction

Osteoporosis (say: "ost-tee-oh-pore-oh-siss") occurs when the inside of the bones become porous from a loss of calcium. This is called losing bone mass. Over time, bones become weak and brittle, which makes them easier to break.

Women are more likely to develop osteoporosis than men. This is due to several factors. Women have less bone mass than men, tend to live longer and take in less calcium. In women, the rate of bone loss speeds up after menopause, when estrogen levels fall. Since the ovaries make estrogen, faster bone loss may also occur if both ovaries are removed by surgery.

Osteoarthritis is the most common type and is more likely to occur as you age. You may feel it in any of your joints, but most commonly in your hips, knees or fingers.

It is recommended that women over 65 years old should have a bone density test / scan.

Risk factors include:
- Alcohol abuse
- Early menopause (before age 45)
- Eating disorders such as anorexia nervosa
- Fair skin (Caucasian or Asian race)
- Family history of osteoporosis
- Hyperthyroidism, either from an overactive thyroid or from taking too much medicine to treat hypothyroidism
- Insufficient calcium
- Long-term use of corticosteroids. These are medicines prescribed to treat inflammation and pain
- Overweight
- Previous injury of the affected joint
- Sedentary lifestyle (not getting enough exercise)
- Smoking or tobacco use
- Surgery to remove ovaries before menopause
- Thin body and small bone frame
- Using the affected joint in a repetitive action that puts stress on that joint (baseball players, ballet dancers, and construction workers are all at risk)

Signs and Symptoms
- Change in posture
- Decrease in height, because osteoporosis can cause your vertebrae (the bones in your spine) to collapse
- Frequent broken bones or fractures
- Low back pain or a hunched back

- A dual-energy X-ray absorptiometry (DEXA). This test measures the density of the bones in your hips, spine, and wrist, which are all places likely to be affected by osteoporosis
- Bone scan
- Computerized Tomography (CT Scan)
- Ultrasound

Treatment(s)

- Dietary changes
- Increase Calcium especially if menopausal
- Increase physical activity

Medication is often prescribed for other long term types of arthritis. Progression can be slowed without medication. Making lifestyle changes without medication is preferable.

## OVA

Introduction

In the female reproductive system the ovaries produce egg cells called ova. The ova is transported to the fallopian tube for fertilization by the sperm, then becomes a fertilised egg.

The fertilized egg is transported to the uterus. Once in the uterus the egg receives the nutrients that it needs for growth and development of the fetus.

# OVARIES

## Introduction

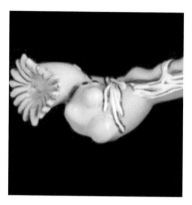

There are two ovaries. One on each side of the uterus and is a part of the female reproductive system. The ova and eggs are produced here.

The ovaries also produce the female hormones known as estrogen and progesterone.

# P

# PAP SMEAR

## Introduction

Papanicolaou smear (Pap smear or Pap test): During a pelvic exam the gynecologist uses a speculum to widen the vagina and swabs the cervix for pre-cancerous and cancerous cells. The Pap smear specimen is sent to a lab.

None of us enjoy placing our feet in those stirrups during the examination, evaluation, and collection of the Pap smear. Stirrups are really for horseback riding, aren't they? But, to get a better view of the vagina it is easier for the gynecologist to have you place your legs in such a position that makes visualization easier. AND, those stirrups never feel comfortable no matter how many times your legs are placed in them.

Early detection of cervical cancer and treatment is best. If your results are normal you should still continue to follow up as indicated by your gynecologist for your annual visit.

If abnormal, your gynecologist will meet with you to discuss your treatment plan.

# PELVIC INFLAMMATORY DISEASE (PID)

## Introduction

PID is a bacterial inflammation of the vagina, cervix, uterus, fallopian tubes and ovaries. This infection is very serious and can leave you sterile.

## Signs and Symptoms
- Bleeding between periods
- Bleeding during intercourse
- Fever
- Nausea
- Pain when passing urine
- Severe abdominal pain and cramps
- Vaginal discharge

It is important to note that some women do not have severe abdominal pain, and PID can go undetected for some time.

## Causes:

PID is most often caused by sexual transmission and it can also be caused by an intrauterine device (IUD). Other causes are douching and other germs that are in the vagina. When PID is diagnosed, the woman's partner must be informed. Men can be silent carriers of the bacteria that causes PID.

PID can recur many times if you are sexually active and / or have multiple sex partners.

## Treatment(s)
- Antibiotics
- Hospitalization

If undetected, you can develop chronic infection and become infertile due to scarring of the fallopian tubes.

# PELVIC ORGAN PROLAPSE

## Introduction

Pelvic organ prolapse is when the pelvic floor muscles weaken and cause some organs to fall downward. These organs are the uterus, vagina, bowel and bladder. Pelvic organ prolapse is not life threatening. By the time most women go to see a doctor the uterus has already fallen into the opening of the vagina.

## Signs and Symptoms
- Bulge near the opening of the vagina
- Difficulty with bowel movement
- Discomfort during sex
- Leak small amounts of urine when you sneeze or cough
- Need to urinate more often
- Not completely emptying the bladder
- Sensation of sitting on a ball
- Sensation of something coming down into the vagina

## Diagnosis
- CT scan of the pelvis
- MRI
- Pelvic examination
- Ultrasound

## Treatment(s)
- Avoid constipation
- Kegel exercises to strengthen the pelvic muscles
- Lose weight
- Medication
- Surgery to repair prolapse
- Vaginal pessary / ring ( a soft, removable device that goes into your vagina)

# PERIMENOPAUSE

## Introduction

Perimenopause is the transitioning period to menopause.

The ovaries make less estrogen. Perimenopause can begin at age 30 to 40 and last until menopause.

The Signs and Symptoms of perimenopause can occur 10 to 15 years before actual menopause, which is the final cessation of your menstrual cycle. Most clinicians will say a woman is postmenopausal once she has not had a period for a year.

The age when the signs of perimenopause occur varies among women. Most women notice perimenopausal signs and symptoms, and some women never have these experiences. The average age for the final menstrual period is 51 years of age.

Women who have had hysterectomies with both ovaries removed usually experience immediate surgical menopause. Women who have had one ovary removed or whose ovaries were left intact experience perimenopause.

## Signs and Symptoms
- Difficulty sleeping, either falling or staying asleep
- Dry skin and / or hair loss
- Heart palpitations (if you experience any heart disturbances, always consult a physician)
- Hot flashes, night sweats, coldness
- Inability to hold your urine
- Irregular periods that can be heavy, light, shorter or longer cycles
- Leaking urine when coughing or sneezing
- Loss of or decreased sexual desire
- Mood changes, anxiety, depression, irritability
- Tender breasts

- Vaginal dryness

There are many other signs and symptoms that women may experience during the perimenopause years. Sometimes perimenopause can be mimicked by other conditions, such as common thyroid disorders. Therefore, it is important that anytime you observe a change in your body dynamics you should consult your physician.

Diagnosis
- Blood test for hormone levels

Treatment(s)
- Birth control pills
- Birth control skin patch
- Decrease alcohol consumption
- Diet
- Exercise
- Progesterone injections
- Stop Smoking
- Vaginal pessary / ring
- Weight Loss

## PREGNANCY

Introduction

Pregnancy in a woman's life can be one of the most fulfilling times in her life. The emotional changes at this time and the numerous questions start: Am I ready to become a mother? Can I afford this child? Would I be able to get rid of my stretch marks? Would I lose the baby weight? How will my lifestyle change?

The physical changes begin, your body begins to look different. There are worries about the ugly stretch marks and the feet as they become swollen. At this time, some women develop the weirdest food cravings.

The good thing about pregnancy is that you are now becoming a mother. As you watch your body change you should enjoy the abdominal changes which reflect the baby's growth. Some women who never had big breasts may now have larger, firmer breasts due to hormonal changes. As your breasts grow make sure that you get a properly fitted bra.

If you are a smoker or drinker, you should stop due to the negative effects on the baby. For example, low birth weight and other health issues. Attend all your prenatal appointments, take prenatal vitamins, and eat the right foods to nourish your body and that of your baby.

It is still important to do mild to moderate exercises with your doctor's approval and you can still have sexual intercourse.

*"Think like a queen. A queen is not afraid to fail. Failure is another stepping stone to greatness."*
Oprah Winfrey

# Q

# Q FEVER

## Introduction

Q fever otherwise known as Query fever is an infection caused by the bacterium Coxiella Burnetii and is exceedingly rare. It affects humans as well as animals. It is mostly spread by animals such as goats, sheep, and cattle. It can be transmitted through sexual contact or through blood transfusions or from a pregnant woman to her fetus. And also by people in occupations such as veterinary medicine, farmers, and animal research.

Causes:  Inhaling dust contaminated by the infected animal feces, urine, or milk

## Signs and Symptoms
- Chills
- Cough
- Diarrhea
- Fatigue / Fever
- Headache
- Muscle aches
- Nausea
- Stomach pain
- Vomiting

## Diagnosis
- Blood test

## Treatment
- Antibiotics
- Supportive care
- Rehydration
- Vaccine

# QUEEN

This book is about women's health and although we could not find many diseases beginning with 'Q,' my sister Stacia who calls herself a 'Queen' suggested that there cannot be a book about women, without an entry on how women should feel about themselves, as 'queens.' We should feel that we are 'queens', treat ourselves as such, and expect others to always treat us as such.

We were finally convinced that because this is really a book on self-care (addressed in another section) this subject should be added. So, we decided to write about a QUEEN. In theory all females are 'queens.' A man might call his wife 'Queen', a son his mother or anyone can affectionately refer to a female as 'Queen'.

The definitions of 'queen' are many such as a 'woman who rules a country', such as Queen Elizabeth II of England, the wife or widow of a King, or a woman who is highly respected in her field such as 'Queen of the Blues.' Calling someone a queen means that the person is held in high regard, or a woman whose name at birth is 'Queen.'

A Queen also is a woman who behaves queenly, who maintains a queenly posture and queenly dignity, speaks with love and kindness; she is quite competent and confident in what she does and always strives to do better and be better. She is secure in her skin, makes no excuses for her authenticity, yet still listens and seeks advice, as necessary.

A woman is considered a queen if she has grit and determination. She is tough, but loving; calm during adversity, is intelligent, loves and knows how to take care of herself.

As women we must always appreciate and love ourselves. After all, we are the only ones who have to live with ourselves, forever. Please pamper yourself, schedule manicures, pedicures and send yourself a subscription of flowers or anything that makes you feel good about yourself. Also, schedule a date night with yourself to have some 'me' time.

While researching the word 'queen' and the meaning of which there are many, I found a book titled *'Queen of Your Own Life'* by Kathy Kinsey and Cindy Ratzlaff. This book lists the 'TOP 10 Ways to Become a Queen' in your own life. I like Number 2, which states that you should *'Place the crown firmly on your head.'*

The book continues that to become a queen all you have to do is to throw a party and there are three mandatory things that should be done (1) you must stand up and in full voice declare yourself queen of your own life, (2) you must do it in front of your trusted friends and give them a chance to do it as well and (3) eat cake. That is, the party cake.

Let us all Embrace ourselves and acknowledge we are all queens, even if it is *"QUEEN FOR A DAY."*


*GO QUEENS!*

# R

# RECTUM

## Introduction

The rectum is the bottom end of the large intestines and is close to the anus. It has little folds. These folds help to keep the stool in place until you need to have a bowel movement. When you are ready, the stool goes into the lower rectum, moves into the anal canal, passes through the anus and leaves the body.

# RHEUMATOID ARTHRITIS

## Introduction

Rheumatoid Arthritis (RA), is an autoimmune disorder. It causes the immune system to attack the joints, which causes painful inflammation. This is a life long condition. Unlike other forms of arthritis like osteoarthritis, RA also attacks the organs like the heart, eyes, and lungs. Of the many forms of arthritis, this is one of the most debilitating types.

Early detection is vital in treating RA because the most damage is done within the first two years. There is no cure or preventative measure for rheumatoid arthritis, there are a number of treatments to alleviate the signs and symptoms.

If RA is not treated, it can lead to permanent joint and bone damage.

## Cause
The cause of RA is unknown, but it can also be an inherited trait.

## Signs and Symptoms
- Fatigue
- Pain
- Physical deformity

- Sensation of pins and needles in the fingers and toes
- Swelling

Diagnosis
- Lab work
- Physical examination

Treatment(s)
- Drink various herbal teas
- Eat a balanced diet
- Eliminate stress
- Have physical therapy
- Regular exercise strengthens the muscles around the joint and increases flexibility
- Surgical options, as recommended by the surgical team. For example, arthroplasty, joint replacement
- There are many things that you can do yourself to make living with the disease easier. While it is tempting to put as little exertion on your sore joints as possible, continue to exercise while avoiding exertion. Perform gentle, slow exercises even during a flare up
- Use heat and cold to ease the pain. Heat should be applied only when the joint is not inflamed, and preferably in the form of a bath or hot shower. Use cold packs on the inflamed joint directly or after strenuous use of the joint
- Work with a rheumatologist to set goals and develop a good treatment plan. Each type of drug has its own side effects. Please make sure that you are informed about the medications that you are taking and report any side effects to your doctor

*"You must love and care for yourself because that's when the best comes out."*
Tina Turner

# S

# SEXUAL INTERCOURSE

## Introduction

The act of the male penis entering the female vagina.

# SEXUALLY TRANSMITTED DISEASES (STD)

## Introduction

There are many diseases that are transmitted sexually such as AIDS, Chlamydia, Herpes, genital warts, gonorrhea, Syphilis, and Trichomoniasis. (Separate sections are available for each disease).

## Treatment(s)
- Practice safe sex
- See your primary care physician for any concerns
- Varies by the disease and usually includes medication

# SNORING

## Introduction

Yes, women do snore! We are embarrassed to admit this, and do not like to be called out on it.

Snoring is a sound from the nose or mouth when breathing is obstructed during sleep. But, after menopause, it may be a sign of sleep apnea. (See sleep apnea).

## Causes
- Alcohol consumption
- Allergy
- Cold
- Menopause
- Nasal congestion

- Obesity
- Structure of the nose

Treatment(s)
- Alcohol avoidance
- Change sleep positions
- Lose weight
- Nasal strips
- Stay hydrated

Diagnosis
- CT scan
- MRI
- Sleep diagnostic study
- X-ray

## SLEEP APNEA

Introduction

Sleep apnea is mainly a disease of men, but women can also be affected during menopause. If you notice that you feel tired during the day or take frequent naps you may have sleep apnea. If your significant other says that you snore loudly and it seems that you gasps for breath during sleep; you need to inform your healthcare professional since you may need to have a sleep diagnostic study.

Signs and Symptoms
- Choking
- Excessive daytime sleepiness
- Fatigue
- Irritability
- Loud breathing

- Snoring
- Sore throat or dry mouth

Treatment
- Lifestyle changes
- Self care (exercise)
- Surgery (for example tonsillectomy, adenoidectomy)
- Weight Loss
- Use of a breathing assistance device at night

## STERILIZATION

Introduction

Sterilization is a woman's inability to have a baby. This can be caused by a disease or a surgical procedure, for example a tubal ligation (tying off of the ovarian tubes); this can be reversed. A disease may result in permanent sterilization.

## SYPHILIS

Introduction

Syphilis is a Sexually Transmitted Disease (STD) caused by direct contact with someone who has an active infection. The germs pass through broken skin or other parts of the body.

Syphilis develops in stages, and Signs and Symptoms vary. If it is not treated it can damage the heart, eyes, brain, spinal cord, bones and joints. This can also cause miscarriage and birth defects.

<u>Signs and Symptoms</u>
- A painless open sore which appears near the vagina after exposure (between 10 days – 3 months)
- Fatigue
- Itching
- Skin rash appears over the body or soles of the feet and palms of the hand
- Swollen lymph nodes
- Vaginal discharge

All might disappear, but the infection remains if not treated.

<u>Treatment(s)</u>
- Antibiotics

*"Strong women don't have 'attitudes', we have standards."*

Marilyn Monroe

# T

# THYROID DISEASE

## Introduction

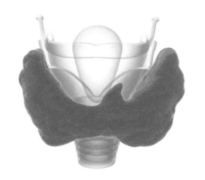

The thyroid gland is one of the largest endocrine glands in the body. It is found in the neck and controls how quickly the body uses energy and makes proteins.

The most common problems of the thyroid gland is that it is either overactive (hyperthyroidism), or underactive (hypothyroidism).

Remember that Graves disease (previously covered) is the most common form of hyperthyroidism.

**Hyperthyroidism** is the overproduction of the thyroid hormones and can increase metabolism.

**Hypothyroidism** is the underproduction of the thyroid hormones and can decrease metabolism. Hashimoto's Hypothyroidism is when the immune system attacks the thyroid gland.

## Signs and Symptoms of *Hyperthyroidism*
Elderly people experience no Signs and Symptoms.
Others may experience the following:
- Depression
- Excessive hunger
- Fatigue
- Irritability
- Panic attacks
- Protrusion or puffy eyes
- Rapid heart beat
- Sweating
- Unexpected weight loss

Treatment(s)

Thyroid hormone treatment is given under the care of a physician and may take a few weeks to become effective.

- Hormone replacement therapy
- Medication
- Radioactive Iodine
- Surgery

Signs and Symptoms of **Hypothyroidism**

- Constipation
- Dry Skin
- Enlarged thyroid
- Fatigue
- Feeling Cold
- Hair Loss
- High cholesterol
- Irritability
- Slow heart rate
- Unexplained weight gain

Treatment(s)

- Medication, under the care of a physician

# TRICHOMONIASIS/ VAGINITIS

## Introduction

Trichomoniasis / Vaginitis is a Sexually Transmitted Disease (STD). If not treated this can cause a bladder infection.

## Signs and Symptoms
- Abdominal pain
- Discomfort during sex
- Heavy, yellow-green or gray vaginal discharge
- Pain when passing urine
- Vaginal itching
- Vaginal odor (fishy)

## Treatment(s)
- Antibiotics

# URINARY PROBLEMS

## Introduction

### 1 – Urinary Incontinence

When stress is placed on the pelvic muscles it is anticipated that you leak urine when coughing, sneezing, laughing, squatting, or lifting something heavy.

### 2 - Overactive bladder

Overactive bladder gives you a strong sudden feeling that you need to urinate. When the muscles in your bladder contract involuntarily. It is possible that you may urinate up to eight times in one day.

### Treatment(s)
- Kegels
- Medications
- Pelvic floor exercises
- Physical therapy
- Vaginal pessary

# URINARY TRACT INFECTION (UTI)

## Introduction

Urinary tract infections (UTI) are caused by germs, usually bacteria that enter the urethra and then the bladder. This can lead to infection, most commonly in the bladder itself, which can eventually spread to the kidneys.

Often your body can get rid of these bacteria, but certain conditions increase the risk of getting a having UTI.

Women tend to get UTIs more often than men because their urethra is shorter and closer to the anus. Because of this, women are more likely to get an infection after sexual activity or when using a diaphragm for birth control. Using a diaphragm can lead to infections because diaphragms push against the urethra and make it harder to completely empty the bladder. When this happens and some urine remains in the bladder, this is likely to grow bacteria and cause infections.

The following also increase your chances of developing a UTI:
- A urinary catheter in place
- Advanced age
- Bowel incontinence
- Diabetes
- Having sex may also cause urinary tract infections in women because bacteria can be pushed into the urethra.
- Kidney stones
- Menopause
- Narrowed urethras, or anything that blocks the flow of urine
- Pregnancy
- Problems emptying your bladder completely (urinary retention)
- Staying still (immobile) for a long period of time
- Surgery or other procedures involving the urinary tract


Signs and Symptoms of a ***bladder infection*** may include:
- Cloudy or bloody urine, which may have a foul or strong odor
- Confusion
- Low fever (not everyone will have a fever)
- Pain or burning with urination
- Pressure or cramping in the lower abdomen (usually middle) or back
- Strong need to urinate often, even right after the bladder has been emptied

Signs and Symptoms of a **_kidney infection_** may include:

If the infection spreads to your kidneys the following are some signs and symptoms:

- Back or groin pain
- Chills
- Confusion (in the elderly, these signs and symptoms often are the only signs of a UTI)
- Fatigue
- Fever above 101 degrees Fahrenheit
- Mental changes
- Nausea and vomiting
- Night sweats
- Severe abdominal pain
- Warm or reddened skin

Exams and Tests

A urine sample is usually collected to perform the following tests:

- Urinalysis – to identify white and red blood cells, bacteria, and to test for certain chemicals, such as nitrites in the urine. Most often, your doctor or nurse can diagnose an infection from the urinalysis report
- Urine culture - clean catch may be done to identify the bacteria in the urine to make sure the correct antibiotic is prescribed for treatment. The term 'clean catch' is when the urine is collected in the following manner
    - clean the area and begin to urinate
    - then stop
    - place a clean cup under your vaginal area and continue to urinate
    - then stop
    - remove the container
    - finish urinating in the toilet bowl
    - follow identified procedure (place cup as instructed)

<u>Treatment(s)</u>
Your doctor must determine the severity of your bladder or kidney infection. Treatment is based on the diagnosis. Antibiotics taken by mouth are usually recommended because there is a risk that the infection can spread to the kidneys. Antibiotics should be taken as prescribed.

It is important that you finish the sequence of antibiotics, even if you feel better. If you do not finish all your antibiotics, the infection could return and may be harder to treat.

Your doctor may also recommend drugs to relieve the burning pain and urgent need to urinate.
Everyone with a bladder or kidney infection should drink plenty of fluids.

Some women may have urinary tract infections that recurs. Such infections are called chronic UTIs. If you have a chronic UTI, you may need antibiotics for many months.

If a structural (anatomical) problem is causing the infection, surgery may be recommended.

A urinary tract infection is uncomfortable, but treatment is usually successful. Relief should come within 24 - 48 hours once treatment begins. If you have a kidney infection, it may take 1 week or longer for relief.

<u>Prevention</u>
Lifestyle changes may help prevent some UTIs.
- After menopause, a woman may choose to use estrogen cream in the vagina area to reduce the chance of further infections.
- Bathing and Hygiene
- Keep your genital area clean

- Take showers instead of baths
- Urinate before and after sexual activity
- Use sanitary pads instead of tampons during menstruation. This is a personal choice. Do the following if using sanitary pads:
    - Avoid bath oils
    - Change pads each time you use the bathroom
    - Clean your genital and anal areas before and after sexual activity
    - Do not douche or use feminine hygiene sprays or powders. It is best to use products that do not contain perfumes in the genital area
- Wipe from front to back after using the bathroom

Clothing
- Avoid tight-fitting pants
- Change underwear and pantyhose at least once a day
- Wear cotton-cloth underwear

Diet
- Do NOT drink fluids that irritate the bladder, such as alcohol and caffeine
- Drink cranberry juice or use cranberry tablets, but NOT if you have a personal or family history of kidney stones
- Drink plenty of fluids

# UTERUS

## Introduction

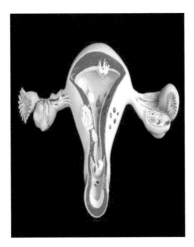

The uterus is a hollow muscular organ in the female pelvis between the bladder and rectum. The upper part of the uterus has the fallopian tubes on both sides, that are open and attached to the ovaries. The lower part of the uterus connects with the vagina.

Ova (eggs) are released from the ovaries and go through the fallopian tubes to the uterus and stay in the uterine walls until prenatal development. The main function of the uterus is to nourish the developing fetus prior to birth.

The uterus changes in size and structure to accommodate the needs of the growing embryo. When the baby is born, the uterus returns almost to its former size.

During menstruation, the uterus is enlarged with increased blood flow. Your period happens when the lining membrane completely disintegrates leading to complete removal through the vaginal opening. At the cessation of menstruation, a fresh membrane is formed.

# UTERINE PROLAPSE

## Introduction

Uterine prolapse is falling or sliding of the uterus from its normal position in the pelvic cavity into the vaginal canal.

## Causes

The uterus is held in position in the pelvis by muscles, special ligaments, and other tissues. If these muscles and connective tissues weaken, the uterus may fall into the vaginal canal (prolapses).

- A pelvic tumor
- Chronic constipation and forced bowel movement
- Chronic cough and obesity which increase the pressure on the pelvic floor
- Lack of or decrease in estrogen hormone after menopause
- Multiple vaginal births
- Normal aging

## Signs and Symptoms

- Difficult or painful sexual intercourse
- Frequent bladder infections
- Frequent urination or a sudden, urgent need to empty the bladder
- Low backache
- Protrusion of the uterus and cervix through the vaginal opening
- Sensation as if sitting on a ball
- Vaginal bleeding or increased vaginal discharge

Many of these signs and symptoms are worse when standing or sitting for long periods of time.

Tests
A pelvic examination performed while the woman is bearing down (as if trying to push out a baby) will show how far the uterus comes down.

The pelvic exam may reveal that the bladder, front wall of the vagina or rectum and back wall of the vagina are entering the vaginal area.

A mass may be noted on the pelvic exam if a tumor is causing the prolapse.

Treatment(s)
Treatment is not necessary unless the signs and symptoms are problematic.
- A vaginal pessary / ring
- Avoid heavy lifting or straining
- Lifestyle changes
- Lose weight if obese
- Surgery, based on signs and symptoms

*"Aging is not" lost youth", but a new stage of opportunity and strength."*

Betty Friedman

# VAGINA

## Introduction

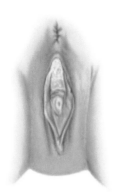

The vagina is an elastic, muscular canal with a soft, flexible lining that provides lubrication and sensation. The vagina connects the uterus to cervix.

The penis enters the vagina during sexual intercourse. The vagina serves as a tunnel for menstrual flow from the uterus. At childbirth, the baby passes through the vagina (birth canal), as the baby is being delivered.

The hymen is a thin, fleshy tissue at the opening of the vagina. It is usually torn during the first sexual encounter, or if something is inserted into the vagina, or ruptured during exercise or accidents.

## VAGINAL PESSARY / RING

### Introduction

A vaginal pessary / ring is a rubber or plastic donut-shaped device that is inserted into the vagina to hold the uterus in place. If there is vaginal prolapse, it may be used as a temporary or permanent form of treatment.

A vaginal pessary is fitted for each individual woman, and can be left in place for up to 3 months. Some pessaries are similar to diaphragms that are used for birth control. Women can be taught how to insert, clean, and remove the pessary / ring.

Some pessaries may interfere with sexual intercourse by limiting the depth of penetration.

Pessaries / rings may cause an irritating and abnormal smelly discharge, and require more frequent cleaning. Occasionally, the pessary / ring may rub on and irritate the vaginal wall, and in some cases may damage the vagina.

If there is a history of uterine prolapse, a woman may wear a pessary / ring by choice, for exercising and other forms of physical therapy; to hold the uterus in place.

Surgery
Surgery should not be done until the prolapse signs and symptoms are worse than the risks of having surgery. The specific type of surgery depends on:
- Degree of prolapse
- Desire for future pregnancies
- Other medical conditions
- The woman's age and general health
- The women's desire to retain vaginal function

Lifestyle Changes
Weight loss is recommended in women with uterine prolapse who are obese.

Heavy lifting or straining should be avoided because they can worsen signs and symptoms.

Coughing can also make signs and symptoms worse. Measures to treat and prevent chronic cough should be tried. If the cough is due to smoking, smoking cessation techniques are recommended.

# VAGINAL PROBLEMS

## Introduction

Vaginal problems are as follows:

Vaginitis: Inflammation of the vagina, commonly from a yeast infection or bacterial overgrowth. Itching, discharge, and change of odor are typical signs and symptoms.

Vaginismus: Involuntary spasm of the vaginal muscles during sexual intercourse. Emotional distress about sex, or medical conditions, can be responsible.

Vaginal warts: Genital warts may affect the vulva or the vagina. Treatments can remove vaginal warts, which are caused by human papillomavirus (HPV).

Vaginal biopsy: In the rare case of a suspicious growth in the vagina, a small piece of tissue (biopsy) may be sent to be checked for cancer.

# VARICOSE VEINS

## Introduction

Normally blood flows in the tiny valves in the veins in the leg, but when the valves lose their functions, the blood that should be moving upward toward the heart pools and presses on the surface vein walls, causing them to bulge. The outcome is swollen, heavy and ugly legs.

Many women who have varicose veins are embarrassed by them since they are unattractive and painful.

Some methods to avoid varicose veins are:
- Avoid long periods of standing
- Diet, if overweight
- Elevate your feet as often as possible
- Stretch frequently when taking long trips such as flying or driving

## Treatment(s)
- Cosmetic removal
- Wear compression stockings

# VIRGINITY

## Introduction

Virginity is the state of being a virgin, a woman who has never had sexual intercourse. The loss of virginity is also the end of being innocent and signals the beginning of sexual activity.

*"Beauty begins the moment you decide to be yourself."*

Coco Chanel

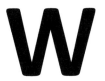

*"Learn to embrace your own unique beauty, celebrate your unique gifts with confidence. Your imperfections are actually a gift."*
Kerry Washington

# THE WOMAN'S BODY

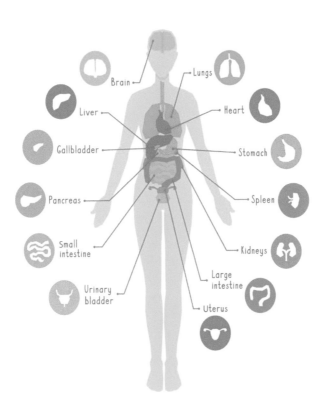

<u>Introduction</u>

*How we view ourselves?*

As women we tend to view ourselves differently. By the color of our skin, the texture of our hair, the shape and size of our bodies and what we wear. Are we too fat, too slim, what do we look like when we walk, when we smile? Is my makeup OK? Is my lipstick the right color or does the lip gloss I have on look good? Am I too short, too tall, too fat, too skinny? Should I relax my hair or leave it natural?

Women generally put too much pressure on themselves to fit in and to look perfect by social norms.

So, we look in the mirror and what do we see? We either see all the faults we can find or a beautiful woman looking back at us.

The faults – nothing looks right. I am too fat, too ugly, my rinse is wearing off and I can see gray hair. My eyes look tired, I have wrinkles on my face, and sun spots. My goodness what is happening?

We try to correct the faults we see. Are they really faults? Are our expectations of ourselves too high? Why not love the person we see staring back at us? No, we go on a binge, dieting, exercising, dying our hair.

Why are we not "comfortable" in our own skins? Is it because of our expectations? Is it the society we live in? Is it cultural? Or, is it all of these?

Let's walk into a room, head held high, well dressed and looking gorgeous. All heads turn, people smile, say how good we look, and the conversation flows.

OR

Let's walk into a room, head down, not well dressed and looking awful. All heads turn, people smirk, says nothing, and the conversation halts.

*What do we prefer?*

So here we go! Each of us must strive to be "comfortable" in our skin because until we get there we are floundering. We are all individuals with individual taste, different income levels and different situations. What we must do is to hold each other up.

Sylvia recalls that many years ago being at a luncheon at her son's school's annual fashion show while sitting at a table with her friends; she looked around the room she saw a woman sitting at a table alone. She immediately approached her and invited her to her table. Her response was," your friends might not want me sitting there." Sylvia responded, "If they are my friends, they will welcome you." She joined Sylvia's table, and they are still very good friends.

*What do we do?*

We should embrace each other. Look out for one another, regardless of skin tones, cultural or differences in body images.

Beauty is in the eyes of the beholder! We are beautiful! Let's celebrate who we are, embrace ourselves and each other. *Laugh*…. those days of self-doubt are behind us.

*"**Hey! Look at me I am a beautiful, gorgeous woman!**"* You should tell yourself this everyday. There is much power in self-talk.

*"And I believe that the best buy in public health today must be a combination of regular physical exercise and a healthy diet."*

Julie Bishop

**(NOTHING BASIC THAT IS UNIQUE TO WOMEN)**

"At the end of the day, your health is your responsibility."

Julian Michaels

# YEAST INFECTION

## Introduction

Yeast infection is caused by a specific type of fungus called Candida albicans. Yeast is commonly present on normal human skin and in areas of moisture, such as the mouth. Also, healthy women normally have yeast in the vagina.

## Causes

Vaginal yeast infections occur when there is an increase in the quantity of yeast already present in the vagina. If you have been previously treated with antibiotics, for any bacterial infection or if you are on immunosuppressive drugs, yeast can multiply and irritate the lining of the vagina.

Vaginal yeast infections can also occur as a result of injury to the inner vagina, such as after chemotherapy.

Other conditions such as diabetes, pregnancy, oral contraceptives, douches or perfumed vaginal hygiene sprays; may also increase a woman's risk of developing a vaginal yeast infection.

A vaginal yeast infection is not considered to be a sexually transmitted infection (STD). Women who are not sexually active can also get a vaginal yeast infection. Women who are sexually active, should inform their sexual partner since his penis can become irritable due to the yeast infection.

## Signs and Symptoms
- Burning
- Itching in the vaginal area
- Pain during intercourse and / or urination
- Soreness
- Vaginal discharge may not be present. If present it is an odorless thick whiteish discharge, and looks like cottage cheese

When a woman has recurring yeast infections of more than four times a year and it is not related to antibiotic use, there might be an underlying medical problem which may require more treatment.

Diagnosis
- Laboratory report from specimen
- Self diagnosed

Treatment(s)
- Antibiotics
- Anti-fungal cream
- Anti-fungal medication
- Drink plenty water
- Modify diet

*"Always be a first-rate version of yourself, instead of a second-rate version of someone else."*

Judy Garland

# Z

(NOTHING BASIC THAT IS UNIQUE TO WOMEN)

**END OF INFORMATIONAL SECTION ON SOME MEDICAL CONDITIONS UNIQUE TO WOMEN**

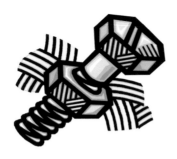

## YOUR BASIC HEALTH MAINTENANCE

### NUTS and BOLTS

In this section of the book, we offer tips to help you work towards a healthier body and lifestyle which includes periodic medical and dental check-ups. We have also included some beauty tips for fun as well as other optional routines that may optimize health and wellbeing.

### HOW TO TALK TO YOUR DOCTOR

Before your appointment do the following:

1. List your questions and concerns
2. Describe your signs and symptoms (tell your doctor what and how you are feeling)
3. Give your doctor a list of your medications, including vitamins and other supplements
4. Be honest about your diet, physical activities, smoking habits, alcohol or drug use
5. Describe any allergies to drugs, food, pollen, or anything else
6. Talk about sensitive topics
7. Ask about tests, procedures and test results, if necessary

8. Tell your doctor if you are pregnant or intend to become pregnant since some medication may not be suitable if pregnant. Also, other prescribed medicine should be used with caution during pregnancy
9. Be sure to discuss all of your concerns before you leave the office. If you do not understand the answer(s) your doctor gives, ask him/her to explain in layman terms
10. Bring a family member or friend you can trust for moral support, to take notes, or in case there is something you might not remember or understand. If your friend or family member is a healthcare professional, that is even better

Getting a Second Opinion:
1. Ask your doctor for a recommendation: do not worry about hurting your doctor's feelings. Most welcome this level of interest in your own health, if not find another doctor
2. Ask someone who you trust for a recommendation
3. Your health insurance carrier may have a list of doctors who provide the services that you may need
4. If you are in the same network and is on a health portal, you can send your medical records, or give access / permission to a new doctor to view your records

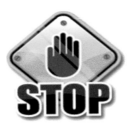

**STOP**

Many women engage in activities that are detrimental to their health, they should consider their health first and everything else falls into place.

STOP:
1. Missing or Skipping meals: Not eating on time or skipping meals leads to a development of gas, ulcers etc.
2. Holding your urine: This is a medium for bacteria. This can lead to stress incontinence, stretched bladder and loss of bladder sensitivity.
3. Holding your stool: This causes the re-absorption of water making the stool hard and difficult to pass.
4. Holding your gas to avoid embarrassment: This is unhealthy and can cause pressure pockets in the colon causing pain and cramping.
5. Douching:  Douching washes away good bacteria in the vagina and can lead to infection. It can also push infection up into the tubules after having sex. This is unnecessary since the vagina cleanses itself.
6. Crossing your legs: This can cause a decrease in circulation. If you really want to cross your legs, then flex your feet often or cross at your ankles.

7. Cutting back on sleep: You may not get sufficient sleep. Too little sleep causes mood swings, leads to stress, memory loss, slows reaction time and affect your metabolism and can cause weight gain.
8. Wearing heels that are too high: You may have a tendency to wear heels that are too high. High heels affect your balance and poor weight distribution, causes cramped toes, bunions and / or corns.

# SOME SIGNS AND SYMPTOMS

## YOU CANNOT AFFORD TO IGNORE

1. Bleeding gums
2. Blurry vision. It may indicate bleeding behind the retina
3. Chest pain
4. Dizziness
5. Headaches that increase in intensity
6. Night sweats
7. Nose bleeds
8. Persistent cough
9. Persistent leg cramps and pain that does not go away
10. Signs of a stroke
    - Drooping mouth
    - Slurred speech
    - Numbness of feet and hands, especially on one side of the body
    - Loss of balance
    - Sudden trouble seeing in one or both eyes
11. Shortness of breath, wheezing and coughing
12. Sudden and increasing pain in the upper right abdomen, especially if you push in on the area and take a deep breath
13. Unexplained weight loss

# TIPS ON THE JOURNEY TO BEAUTY

We will document the daily, weekly, monthly, quarterly and annual steps you should take. These are suggestions only. Some are homemade or easy to use products. We are not endorsing any products or suggesting that our choices are the only ones.

## Bathing/Showering

To keep skin moist it is best to use skin cleansers or soap with Kaolin for bathing or showering. The water should be warm (not hot), lather skin well and apply body oil to damp skin (if desired).

## Body Scrub

This can be done as often as you like and it helps to remove dead skin. After the scrub, a full body moisturizer should be applied to give your skin a soft supple feeling. Treat yourself either monthly or every three months by going to a spa to have this done (See "The Spa" in the Monthly section).

Many people are using skin products with Shea butter these days since reports state that it is one of the best ingredients for use in most skin and hair products.

# BEAUTY TIPS

## FACE

Daily routine
- If you wear makeup use sparingly and wisely
- Moisturize
- Tone
- Wash

Use the product of your choices

Nightly routine
- Wash
- Apply night cream
- Remove makeup before going to bed. The danger of constantly wearing make-up and sleeping in it creates blocked pores. Makeup can be removed with olive oil around the eyes or nonabrasive cleaners.
- Tone
- Use eye cream if you wish

Twice a week
Exfoliate face, hands, lips, and heels. This helps to remove dead skin.

Weekly
Facial (could be a home facial, please see below).

Every six weeks
Treat yourself to a salon facial.
Here are some home facial recipes:

Simplicity at its best:

- Blend oatmeal, cornmeal, avocado, milk, lime juice, olive oil, and honey to a thick paste. Apply to face; leave on 5-10 minutes. Rinse with lukewarm, then cool water. If you mix too much you can easily refrigerate the excess. It feels nice and cool when it is applied directly from the fridge. (Sylvia's preference is the homemade facial masks).
- Mix 2 egg whites with a few drops of lemon juice. Apply; leave on for 5-7 minutes then rinse. (As the eggs dry, they tighten the skin and pull debris out of the pores. Lemon helps to exfoliate).

For cleaning pores- use a sugar scrub

- Mix 1 tablespoon each of sugar, lemon juice, olive oil, and honey. Wet face, apply scrub, and rub gently in a circular motion. Remove with warm wet washcloth, then rinse.
- Squeeze lemon or lime onto ice cube. Rub over face, the natural acids gently exfoliate.

Fountain of youth cocktail:

- Mix a tablespoon of honey with avocado and apply to the face for 1 minute, then cleanse face with cool water (this is good for wrinkles).
- Put oatmeal in cold water, place washcloth in the water, squeeze washcloth and apply/hold to your face for 1 minute.

Oatmeal is supposed to be very good for sensitive skin and it tightens pores.

*These days you can purchase an already prepared face masks – this is a moist cloth face covering with cut outs for the eyes, nose, and lips. They come in different types and are very easy to use. This is a our new fad. We never forget this weekend "ritual."*

*We recommend that our sisters have at least a weekly facial, even if homemade.*

**HAIR**

Shampoo as often as you feel it is necessary with a shampoo of your choice. We recommend shampoos with Panthenol. A good conditioner is an important aspect of hair grooming. One of our friends rinses her hair with Rosemary and sleeps overnight with it in her hair as a conditioner. This is something she learned from her grandmother.

# PERIODIC CHECK-UPS
# &
# TREATMENTS

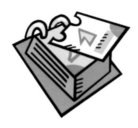

**DAILY**

Teeth
- Brush teeth 2-3 times daily
- Floss at night or anytime you choose to do so
- Gargle with mouthwash

Hands
- Keep your hand soft and conditioned with a good hand cream or lotion
- Wash hands often, and especially after using the bathroom

Makeup
- Apply sparingly

Before bed:
- Wash face
- Apply night cream to face
- Remove makeup
- Tone face
- Use eye cream if you wish

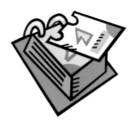

**WEEKLY**

<u>Body and Face</u>
Exfoliate body or face with a buffing cream
- Wash using a cleansing gel (preferably)

<u>Finger and Toe nails</u>
- Apply polish of your choice
- Do manicure at home or at salon
- If diabetic see a podiatrist
- Should be kept short and clean

<u>Heels</u>
- Do pedicure at home or at salon
- Exfoliate or buff your heels, and apply a heel cream or lotion of choice
- If diabetic see a podiatrist

<u>Lips</u>
Exfoliate lips weekly (Use either a store bought exfoliant or simple sugar)

<u>Shaving and Hair removal</u>
- Shave legs and underarms, using cream and / or razors.

<u>Manicures and Pedicures</u>
- Weekly or bi-weekly can help to keep your nails in good condition.

<u>Waxing</u>

- Be very careful when doing a self wax. The first time I tried this at home, I cried as I removed the wax because I had applied the wax to the entire leg instead of one section at a time. Of course I never did my other leg, and needless to say I have not tried this at home since. (Sylvia's account).
- Eyebrows, lips, cheek, and chin.   We both hate to have our lips waxed.
- Only perform self waxing if you are good at it and follow instructions carefully. Many women tend to use depilatory creams, but that is a matter of choice.
- Under arms and Legs
- Personal choice, when indicated

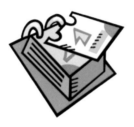

**MONTHLY**

<u>Massage</u>

Monthly (either at home or at a salon), a good body massage relieves stress, and muscle aches and pains.

<u>The Spa</u>

What luxury! Spending a day at a spa in a fluffy robe, and slippers without a care in the world is wonderful. Half way through the day, a simple healthy meal is provided. You can go alone or with a group of friends. Betty and I prefer to go away for a weekend retreat with a group of girlfriends and luxuriate in having facials, manicures, pedicures, body scrubs, and mud wraps. The hot tub and massages complete the day.

It is a good idea to get to the spa early, and spend 15 minutes in the steam room, have a glass of water, a cup of tea and eat some fruit as you relax before your session begins.

At the end of the day you leave floating on air and rejuvenated. Enjoy!

This experience can be monthly or whenever you feel that you deserve to treat yourself or be treated. Do not wait for birthdays, anniversaries, or Mother's Day.

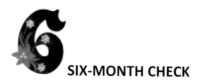

**SIX-MONTH CHECK**

## SIX-MONTH CHECK
- Dental visit
- Follow up as indicated by your Primary Care physician or specialist.

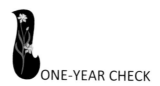

ONE-YEAR CHECK

## ONE-YEAR CHECK
- Eye examination
- Follow up as indicated by your Primary Care physician or specialist.
- Full physical examination with your Primary Care Physician
- Gynecologist for Pap smear, manual breast and abdominal examinations
- Mammogram
- Sonogram / Ultrasound

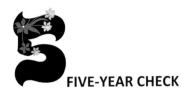 **FIVE-YEAR CHECK**

## FIVE-YEAR CHECK

- After the initial colonoscopy baseline is done at age 45 (earlier if indicated.) This is usually repeated every five (s) years. If polyps are removed during the colonoscopy, a repeat may be done in 3 years. Your doctor will inform you of the frequency.

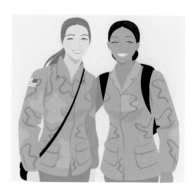

## GIRLFRIENDS

We cannot end this instructional and informational guide without addressing the joy of having girlfriends.

Having girlfriends to spend time with is very important. It creates a bond that is very difficult to break. Girlfriends are there through thick and thin and are your confidantes. We are "Girlfriends" and are part of a group called Les Chausettes. We meet as often as possible, have girlfriends get to-gathers, pyjama parties, movie dates, attend dinners and shows in the city, and are planning to take a cruise with the full group. Betty and I took one together a few years ago. It was as "girlfriends", and sister-nurses that Betty and I decided to write this book.

It has been well documented that having this bond with a group of friends helps in many extraordinary ways.

Connecting frequently through phone calls, arranged meetings, weekly or monthly, at one another's home, taking vacations together and Spa outings is an actual part of the bonding experience.

Girlfriends are there through marriages, divorces, death or other stages of each other's lives. They are the ones you turn to when things are bad, when things are good or if you even want a good cry or a sounding board. You can share things without being embarrassed. Girlfriends know your likes and dislikes and can even "read" your mind with just a glance.

Having this deep-rooted bond helps to inspire and challenge you, and helps to make life more worthwhile. It does not matter how many girlfriends you have, what is important is the quality of those friendships.

Having a best friend or friends enables you to pursue your goals and dreams knowing that you not only have strong support, but people who will give their honest opinion, feedback, and guidance. If you are close to others it also helps you to have a special feeling of self- worth and view life from a more positive angle. Having a few good friends with whom you can discuss anything, makes you happier and more at peace with yourself and the world.

**SPENDING TIME WITH MY FAVORITE PERSON**

# ME

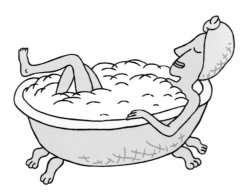

Weekly Tub Time / Spending time with ME

Each of us need some alone time.

Some of the things that accompany ME when spending time with myself are:

- Scented Candle
- Glass of wine
- Soft music
- Bubble bath
- Bath Oils
- Dim lights
- Do not take phone to the bathroom

***Relax and enjoy, but do not fall asleep. If you are feeling drowsy or sleepy leave the tub.***

# SOME HELPFUL CONTACT INFORMATION

Alcoholics Anonymous
www.aa.org
1-888-964-4572

American Association
of Kidney Patients
https://aakp.org
1-800-749-2257

American Cancer Society
www.cancer.org
1-800-227-2345

American Diabetes Association
www.diabetes.org
1-800-342-2383

American Heart Association
www.heart.org
1-800-242-8721

Arthritis Foundation
www.arthritis.org
1-800-283-7800

Eating Disorder
www.eatingdisorders.org
1-888-510-6145

Lupus Support Group
www.lupus.org
1-800-558-0121

Substance Abuse and Mental
Health Services Administration
(SAMHSA)
www.samhsa.gov
1-800-662-4357

Suicide Prevention
www.suicidepreventionlifeline.org
1-800-273-8255

The Obesity Society
www.obesity.org

**"A woman is like a tea bag- you never know how strong she is until she gets in hot water."**

Eleanor Roosevelt

**"My mother told me to be a lady. And for her, that meant be your own person, be independent."**

Ruth Bader Ginsburg

# REFERENCES

A.D.A.M., Inc. is accredited by URAC, also known as the American Accreditation HealthCare Commission (www.urac.org). URAC's accreditation program is an independent audit to verify that A.D.A.M. follows rigorous standards of quality and accountability. A.D.A.M. is among the first to achieve this important distinction for online health information and services. Learn more about A.D.A.M.'s editorial policy, editorial process, and privacy policy. A.D.A.M. is also a founding member of Hi-Ethics and subscribes to the principles of the Health on the Net Foundation (www.hon.ch).

About.com.AIDS/HIV. Retrieved 5/13/2011 from http://www. aids.about.com/od/hivtesting/a/hivdiag.htm

American Diabetes Association
https://www.diabetes.org
(800) 342-2383

American Heart Association
https://www.heart.org
(800) 242-8721

Anorexia>
Http://www.mayoclinic.com/health/anorexia/sinD500606.
Retrieved Aug 18,2011

Arthritis Foundation
https://www.arthritis.org

AllRefer.Comhealth
http:wwwhealth.allrefer.com/health

Bulima
Bulimia:www.webmd.com. RETRIEVED June 10,2013
Bulmia:www.nlm.nih.gov/medlineplus/ency/article/100341.htm.
Retrieved June 10,2013

Cornforth, Tracey. Are you depressed? About.com Guide. Updates October 30, 2009. Retrieved 3/10/12 from http://www.about.com

Denise Foley, Eileen Nechas and the Editors of Prevention Magazine. Women's Encyclopedia of Health and Emotional Healing. Top Women Doctors Share Their Unique Self-Help Advice on Your Body, Your Feelings and Your Life. Rodale Press. Emmaus, Pennsylvania1993

Douching: The Doctor/v show. Lisa Masterson"The Vagina is a self cleaning oven"

Douching http://www.women,webmd.com/vagina-douching. Retrieved Aug 19,2011

Eczema: www.nationaleczema.org/living-with-eczema-quick-fact-sheet. Retrieved July 13,2013

Emedicinehealth- Retrieved on 5/13/12 from http://www.emedicinehealth.com/genital_warts/pages5_em.htm .

Endocrine Glands: Wikipedia retrieved data  7/7/13 http://en.wikipedia.org/wiki/Endocrine_gland

Fighting Fibroids: Essence Magazine:May 2014

Food Pyramid

Graig's Anatomy of the Human Body.XL. Splanchnology

https://www.cdc.gov/diabetes/prevention/oindex.html CDC-Centers for Disease Control and Prevention. Retrieved July 31,2018National Institute of Diabetes and Digestive and Kidney Diseases. Retrieved on July 31, 2018,Https://www.niddk.nih.gov/health-information/diabetes/overview/preventing-problems/foot-problems

https://www.fns.usda.gov/mypyramid

http://www.nhs.uk/conditions/Pages/bodymap.aspx?Index=A

https://www.cdc.gov>gov>qfever

https://www.clevelandclinic.org>health

https://www.mayoclinic.org>q-fever

Healthdirect, Female Reproductive System. Retrieved June/5/2019

Kimmey M.B. Complications of gastrointestinal endoscopy. In: Feldman M, Friedman LS, Brandt LJ, eds. Sleisenger and Fordtran's Gastrointestinal and Liver Disease. 9th ed. Philadelphia, Pa: Saunders Elsevier; 2010: chap

Lupus.Lupus.org/newsite/index.html. Retrieved June 22,2013

MedicineNet.com (Yeast Infection). Retrieved May 30.2012 fr(Medicinet.com/script/main/forum.asp?articlekey=24728)

http:www.medicinenet.com/yeast_vaginitis/article.hlm.

MedlinePlus- The trusted Health Information for You.

Mittelschmerz (Painful Ovulation)

MyClevelandclinic.org/disorders/mihelschmerz/hic_mittelschmerz _painful_ovulation.aspx. Retrieved June 22, 2013.

Obesity www.webmd.com/diet/what_is_obesity. Retrieved March 10, 2012

Oz, Emmett, M.D, Host of The Dr. Oz show ( Fox Channel 5)

Organ Donation https://www.organdonor.gov

Pasricha P, J. Gastrointestinal endoscopy. In: Goldman L, Ausiello D, eds. Cecil Medicine. 23rd ed. Philadelphia, Pa: Saunders Elsevier; 2007:chap 136.Update Date: 11/23/2010

PubMed Health is a consumer health Web site produced by the National Center for Biotechnology Information (NCBI), a division of the National Library of Medicine (NLM) at the National Institutes of Health (NIH). PubMed Health provides up-to-date information on diseases, conditions, injuries, drugs, supplements, Treatment options, and healthy living, with a special focus on comparative effectiveness research from institutions around the world.

Pubmed.Health http://www.ncbr.nlm.nih.gov/pubmedhealth/PMH0002477

*What are the signs of heart attack in women? Excerpt taken from"*
*Meet your heart. Oprah Magazine. Dr. Mehmet Oz. February*
*2011. Oprah.com*

*Parents' Magazine's Self-Guidance Program To Successful*
*Parenthood. Published by Parents'Magazine Enterprises.*

*Queen of Your Own Life: The Grown-Up Woman's Guide to*
*Claiming Happiness and Getting the Life You Deserve by Kathy*
*Kinsey and Cindy Ratzlaff*

*The Signs and Symptoms of Perimenopause*

*From Tracee Cornforth, former About.com Guide updated*
*September 04, 2009*

*Retrieved March 10, 2012*

*Thyroid Gland. En.wikipedia.org/wiki/Thyroid. Retrieved June 22,*
*2013*

*Updated by: David C. Dugdale, III, MD, Professor of Medicine,*
*Division of General Medicine, Department of Medicine, University*
*of Washington School of Medicine; and George F. Longstreth, MD,*
*Department of Gastroenterology, Kaiser Permanente Medical Care*
*Program, San Diego, California. Also reviewed by David Zieve, MD,*
*MHA, Medical Director, A.D.A.M., Inc.*

*Women's Health Calendar (2008) US Department of Health and*
*Human Services: Office of Women's Health.*
*http://www.womenshealth.gov*

*WebMD: Digestive Disorders Health Center. Article Link HTTP://*
*www.. webmd.com/digestive-disorders/picture-of-the-*
*colonhttp://www.nhs.uk/conditions/Pages/bodymap.aspx?Index=*
*A*

*Your Urinary Tract: A User's Manual. Health Magazine( May*
*2014.)*

# EPILOGUE

*The ABCs of Women's health is all about the basics of the female body, keys to maintaining health, and information about the illnesses unique to women. As veteran nurses with over 70 years of combined experience in health care, authors Sylvia M. Barchue and Betty L. Gadson only became aware of most of what they are sharing with their readers once they entered the medical field. This gives you, the reader, more leverage and knowledge for self care and caring for loved ones than Sylvia and Betty had before gaining expertise. In addition to preventative and self care, they strongly advocate a close collegial partnership between you, your doctors and other health care providers. Such a partnership serves to optimize your health results and ultimately improve your quality of life. Please, read this book for yourself and remember to purchase copies for the women in your lives. "The ABCs of Women's Health- What Every Woman Needs to Know". To me this title is appropriate. Growing up as a child and young woman in the Caribbean I was aware that I had the following: eyes, nose, ears, hair, mouth, lips, breasts, hands and feet, but what else? I had a tummy, a vagina, and oh a head and a neck.*

*I had no idea what was inside of the frame that was me, and apart from measles and chicken pox I knew of no other disease or illnesses, and yes occasionally I heard that someone had the secret and dreaded disease- CANCER.*

*It was only when I went to nursing school in London that I learned that there is so much more a woman needs to know about herself. A few years ago I began toying with the idea of writing a simple to understand book. Suddenly, one day I knew what the title would be and I actually told Betty that she would write this book with me. In partnership we have put together a book which includes knowledge, fun and healthy activities.*

*Thank you to all the young ladies and women who read this book and take actions to better your health. We own our bodies, and we must take care of them.*

*In health,*

*Sylvia.*


*I am a Registered Nurse whose passion for helping people led to a satisfying career in nursing. I enjoy teaching and helping to write this book has fulfilled a lifelong dream of publishing. Thanks to the help and encouragement of my friend Sylvia, I finally did.*

*It is my wish that you find this book helpful. And discuss solutions with your health care providers to assist you to restore and maintain good health.*

*In health,*

*Betty.*

# CO-AUTHORS

SYLVIA M. BARCHUE, MS, RN, a retired Registered Nurse 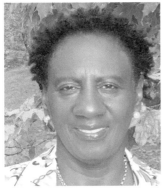 executive and highly effective leader, earned her nursing Diploma, London, England; a BA in Leadership (Magda cum Laude) from Sacred Heart University, Fairfield, CT; an MS in Organization and Management with specialization in Leadership (Summa cum Laude) from Capella University, Minneapolis, MN; a Certificate in Nursing Management, Fairfield University, CT; and, is a graduate of the North East Healthcare Leadership Institute with Distinction as the first Veterans Health Administration Fellow Mentor at James J. Peters, VAMC, Bronx, NY; also a first for all VHAs. She has published and collaborated on books and medical journal articles.

BETTY L. GADSON, RN, a retired Registered Nurse with 41 years of 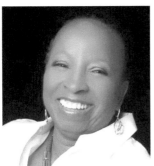 experience in multiple areas of clinical and administrative nursing. Her career in the field of Health Care helped to fuel her passion for preventative and wholistic medicine. In addition to her many studies in clinical medicine she developed a keen interest in research in the area of the improvement of health through diet, nutrition, herbal, supplemental therapies and other natural practices. This is her first experience co-authoring a book.